陶敏芳 主审

盆底的科学
解除盆底功能障碍的缄默密约

[澳] 彼得·佩特洛斯　帕特里夏·斯奇琳　琼·麦克格蕾迪 著

吴氢凯 滕银成 薛卓维 主译

U0295434

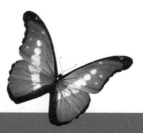

基于盆底整体理论，帮助全球数百万女性重拾希望

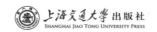

上海交通大学出版社
SHANGHAI JIAO TONG UNIVERSITY PRESS

内容提要

本书介绍了盆底器官及其韧带的解剖结构、生理功能，并用插图和漫画形象地解释了盆底器官脱垂和功能失调的病因与治疗方法。书中结合了众多真实患者的病例故事和心路历程，将"整体理论"相关的基础知识和临床应用娓娓道来，通俗易懂，力图鼓励有着相同症状的女性勇敢地面对疾病，打破沉默，重拾希望。

图书在版编目(CIP)数据

盆底的科学：解除盆底功能障碍的缄默密约/(澳)彼得·佩特洛斯(Peter Petros)，(澳)帕特里夏·斯奇琳(Patricia M Skilling)，(澳)琼·麦克格蕾迪(Joan McCredie)著；吴氢凯，滕银成，薛卓维主译. —上海：上海交通大学出版社，2023.9

ISBN 978-7-313-22624-2

Ⅰ.①盆… Ⅱ.①彼…②帕…③琼…④吴…⑤滕…⑥薛… Ⅲ.①女性—骨盆底—功能性疾病—治疗 Ⅳ.①R711.5

中国版本图书馆 CIP 数据核字(2019)第 255668 号

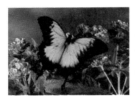

尤利西斯蝴蝶(蓝山蝴蝶)，仅生存于昆士兰州北部地区
它象征着"整体理论系统"的应用缓解了本书所列举的女性疼痛和失禁症状，使她们重塑身心，这也是本书的精华所在。

盆底的科学——解除盆底功能障碍的缄默密约
PENDI DE KEXUE——JIECHU PENDI GONGNENG ZHANG'AI DE JIANMO MIYUE

著　者：	[澳]彼得·佩特洛斯(Peter Petros) [澳]帕特里夏·斯奇琳(Patricia M Skilling) [澳]琼·麦克格蕾迪(Joan McCredie)	主　译：	吴氢凯 滕银成 薛卓维	
出版发行：上海交通大学出版社		地　址：上海市番禺路 951 号		
邮政编码：200030		电　话：021-64071208		
印　制：上海锦佳印刷有限公司		经　销：全国新华书店		
开　本：850mm×1168mm　1/32		印　张：7.25		
字　数：176 千字				
版　次：2023 年 9 月第 1 版		印　次：2023 年 9 月第 1 次印刷		
书　号：ISBN 978-7-313-22624-2				
定　价：98.00 元				

编译委员会名单

原 著：Peter Petros，Patricia M Skilling，Joan McCredie
主 译：吴氢凯　滕银成　薛卓维
主 审：陶敏芳

参 译：（按姓氏笔划排序）

王建六　北京大学人民医院
方伟林　上海交通大学医学院附属仁济医院
吕坚伟　上海交通大学医学院附属仁济医院
田维杰　中国医学科学院北京协和医院
朱 兰　中国医学科学院北京协和医院
李 洁　上海交通大学医学院附属第六人民医院
李 毓　上海交通大学医学院附属第六人民医院
李松芳　北京大学人民医院
刘 斌　上海交通大学医学院附属第六人民医院
刘梦宇　上海交通大学医学院附属第六人民医院
邱 雨　上海交通大学医学院附属第六人民医院
张 睿　上海交通大学医学院附属第六人民医院
张晓薇　广州医科大学附属第一医院
陈立奇　上海交通大学医学院附属第六人民医院
周月娣　上海交通大学医学院附属第六人民医院
徐 玮　上海交通大学医学院附属第六人民医院
徐依赟　上海交通大学医学院附属第六人民医院
黄程胜　上海交通大学医学院附属第六人民医院
梁 爽　上海交通大学医学院附属第六人民医院
梁早雪　广州医科大学附属第一医院

Publish information

Obstructive defecation
Fecal incontinence
Pelvic Organ Prolapse

A guide for symptom relief with illustrative patient stories.

Based on the Integral Theory System which has already helped millions of women worldwide with stress urinary incontinence

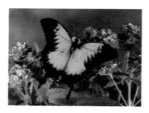

Ulysses or Mountain Blue Butterfly is found only in Northern Queensland.

It symbolizes the freedom which the women described in this book experienced when their burden of pain and incontinence was lifted by application of the Integral System method, the substance of this book.

出版说明

排便障碍
粪失禁
盆腔器官脱垂

帮助患者症状缓解、心路释然的科学指南

基于让全球数百万压力性尿失禁患者已然受益的"整体理论系统"

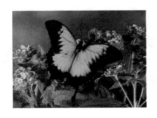

尤利西斯蝴蝶(蓝山蝴蝶),仅生存于昆士兰州北部地区

它象征着"整体理论系统"的应用缓解了本书所列举女性的疼痛和失禁症状,使她们重塑身心,也是本书的精华所在

译者序

　　2007 年,南太平洋一只蓝色的蝴蝶振翼飞向上海,中国妇产科同仁从此认识了"整体理论"。女性盆底"整体理论"由澳大利亚妇科泌尿专家 Peter Petros 教授和瑞典的 Ulmsten 教授于 1990 年首次提出,是一个集解剖、肌电生理、影像检查、临床诊断和手术治疗于一体的理论体系。2007 年 9 月,《女性骨盆底——基于整体理论的功能、功能障碍及治疗》第二版的中文版由上海市第六人民医院(上海交通大学医学院附属第六人民医院)罗来敏教授团队翻译,上海交通大学出版社出版发行。该书将复杂隐秘的盆底解剖付诸于形象生动的模拟图形,使其描述的理论和医学哲学浅显易懂。自"整体理论"引入中国以来,我国的盆底事业蒸蒸日上,盆底整体重建的理念已被广泛接受。

　　今年,我们再度翻译 Peter Petros 教授的患者教育手册 *Unlocking the Female Pelvic Floor*,以中英文对照的形式,由上海交通大学出版社出版发行。本书共分 10 章,由 Peter Petros 教授、Patricia Skilling 和 Joan McCredie 撰写。分别介绍膀胱、子宫、直肠以及其功能,阴道或其韧带的损伤如何导致这些器官的疾病,治疗方案的选择以及通过具体的就诊经历解除患者的顾虑。书中有诸多真实患者的病例,作者用简明的语言阐述了盆底疾病的发病机制和基于"整体理论系统"的治疗方法。本书的精髓是:从尿频、尿急、漏尿、夜尿、便秘、阴道块物脱出、下腹疼痛、性交疼痛等盆底功能障碍性疾病的症状出发,通过抽丝剥茧的方式,推导出可能存在的盆底解剖缺陷,并用整体的理念加以修复，从而改善或治愈疾病。尿道中段悬吊术治疗压力性尿失禁就是应用本书原理的典型范例，目前已经给全球数百万患者带来了福音。但读者也必须认识到，盆底功能障碍的病因是极其复杂的，相同的症状可由多种病因所致。盆底支持组织松弛只是其中的一个病因，单纯加强盆底组织支持并不能完全缓解所有症状。针对盆底功能障碍性疾病高发病率、低就诊率的现状，作者鼓励患者抛开自卑，勇敢地面对疾病，寻求治愈——解除患者"保持缄默的密约"。目前，本书已在德国、意大利、罗马尼亚、美国以及拉丁美洲的多个国家出版发行，其核心理念也被世界许多国家的医生所接受。

本书适合盆底功能障碍性疾病的患者以及妇产科、泌尿科、肛肠科、整形科的各级医生阅读。浅显易懂的中文译文也适合患者阅读。对于盆底诊疗感兴趣的各科医生而言，中英文对照的形式，也对其提高专业英语能力、更好地理解原著的精髓大有裨益。由于本书是中英文对照，翻译中肯定存在不妥或错误之处，敬请各位读者、同行不吝赐教，在此衷心感谢！

感谢澳大利亚 Peter Petros 教授无私地授予我们中文版版权。感谢中国医学科学院北京协和医院妇产科朱兰教授、北京大学人民医院妇产科王建六教授、广州医科大学附属第一医院妇产科张晓薇教授、上海交通大学医学院附属仁济医院泌尿科吕坚伟主任在百忙之中参与本书的翻译工作。翻译过程也得到了上海交通大学出版社以及医学分社王华祖社长的大力支持，上海交通大学医学院附属第六人民医院妇产科的翻译团队承担了大量的翻译和审校工作，在此一并表示感谢！

让我们共同祝愿我国的女性盆底事业不断发展壮大！

译者

2021 年 11 月 16 日于上海

作者介绍

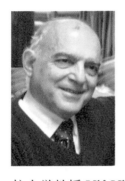

彼得·佩特洛斯（Peter Petros）教授，科学博士（西澳大利亚大学），哲学博士（乌普萨拉大学），医学学士、科学学士、医学博士（悉尼）、英国皇家妇产科学院荣誉院士（伦敦），是一位经验丰富的盆底重建外科医生。在尿失禁和脱垂领域的基础研究和临床手术方面，他是国际公认的引领者。20世纪90年代初，他和已故的瑞典乌普萨拉大学教授 Ulf Ulmsten 发明了治疗压力性尿失禁的尿道中段悬吊手术。这种创新术式基于 Petros 和 Ulmsten 教授革命性的整体理论，该理论也是本书的基石。自2000年以来，全世界至少施行了150万例此类手术。Petros 教授撰写了170多篇有关尿失禁和脱垂的原创性科学论文，并在悉尼新南威尔士大学（University of NSW，Sydney）、美国凯斯西储大学（Case Western Reserve University）、美国俄亥俄州克利夫兰医学中心（Cleveland，Ohio）担任医学教授，在西澳大利亚大学（University of Western Australia）担任工程学教授。他撰写的《女性骨盆底》这一重要医学书籍，现在已是第三版，被翻译成8种语言。Petros 教授现生活和工作在悉尼。

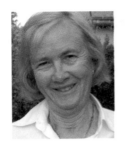

帕特里夏·斯奇琳(Patricia Skilling)医生，医学学士、外科学学士(毕业于英国圣安德鲁斯大学)，师从 Petros 教授。作为 Kvinno 中心的盆底康复(Pelvic Floor Rehabilitation，PFR)总监，她开创了整体理论盆底康复系统。这是自 1948 年 Kegel 运动疗法后，第一个全新的治疗系统。她的相关研究成果发表在重要的科学期刊上。该新系统具有时效性高的特点，同时改善了 Kegel 方法无法解除的许多症状，例如尿急、夜尿、盆腔疼痛、排尿异常以及压力性尿失禁等。

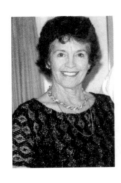

琼·麦克格蕾迪(Joan McCredie)，具有 25 年尿失禁治疗和舒缓治疗的经验。作为倡导者，她曾多次为妇女团体和民间组织演讲。作为诊所的顾问，她与 Petros 教授和 Skilling 医生合作密切。她对失禁和疼痛可能对女性生活造成深刻心理影响的同情、理解和关注，对患者和医生的工作都是无价的。

(上海交通大学医学院附属第六人民医院妇产科，刘梦宇 译，吴氢凯 校)

A CONSPIRACY OF SILENCE

I write from my own personal experience as a woman who had the problem of severe chronic pelvic pain and incontinence and who had to face the fact that I needed to seek professional advice. Later, as a staff member of the first clinic in the world based on the methods outlined in this book, I had the opportunity to observe and discuss with other women, how their bladder, bowel and pain problems had affected not only their quality of life but also, the very essence of their being.

What I heard, confirmed the opinion I had formed, that the subject of incontinence has been hidden away by generations of women, a passive conspiracy of silence. During my time at the clinic, I realized that there is no age group that is untouched. It occurs even in children, in younger women during sport, during pregnancy and after childbirth. But incontinence is about much more than just the mechanics of bladder and bowel function which are described in this book. For the individual sufferer, it is a powerfully emotive issue. It causes acute embarrassment, erosion of self-confidence and self-esteem. Even the least fastidious woman knows that an odour could be perceptible to others in her company. This leads to a reluctance to socialize, which in turn further depletes her self-image. She has to cope with a high level of constant anxiety, such as having to be aware of the location of toilets. Some addressed their fate with resignation, others with bitterness.

缄默的密约

本书源自我的亲身经历,作为一名女性,面对严重的慢性盆腔疼痛和大小便失禁,我不得不寻求专业的帮助。后来,我成为了世界上第一家基于本书理论而设立的诊所的工作人员。我有幸与一些有类似经历的女性患者进行交流,进而认识到膀胱、肠道和疼痛问题不仅影响着她们的生活质量,还影响着她们的生活信念。

我的见闻证实了我的观点,那就是,自古以来,女性对于失禁的话题总是避而不谈,就像是一种消极的"保持缄默的密约"。在诊所工作期间,我发现所有年龄段的女性都受此困扰,甚至包括儿童,以及运动中、怀孕期和产后的年轻女性。但事实上,失禁的发生机制远不止本书所述的膀胱和肠道功能受损那么简单。对具体患者而言,它还是一个强烈的情感问题。它让人非常尴尬,对自信和自尊也是一种摧残。因为即使是最不在意的女性,也会意识到工作单位中的其他人可能会察觉到某种异味。这导致她不愿社交,自我形象进一步受损。更让人难堪的是,她往往非常焦虑,例如必须明确知晓厕所的位置。为此,一些人选择听天由命,另一些人则苦不堪言。

Many patients who came to our clinic had already exhausted all standard avenues of treatment. They were recommended because it offered them hope of cure for conditions which had been considered incurable.

We have written this book for the woman who needs to understand how her pelvic organs work and how and why the methods so successfully applied by physicians who follow the new system promise to be a major step in finally lifting the veil of this conspiracy of silence.

Joan McCredie

　　许多患者在来我们诊所就诊之前,已经尝试过所有能想到的方法。她们之所以慕名而来,是因为我们诊所为这些已经被判为无可救药的患者提供了治愈的希望。

　　我们之所以为这些女性患者编写此书,是想帮助她们了解盆腔器官的工作机制,以及遵循新治疗系统的医生如何治愈此类患者,该系统的应用将成为揭开缄默密约面纱的重要一步。

琼·麦克格蕾迪

(上海交通大学医学院附属第六人民医院妇产科,刘梦宇 译,吴氢凯 校)

Foreword—What is different about this book?

By Dr Bernhard Liedl, President, ICOPF (International Collaboration of Pelvic Floor Surgeons) Munich, Germany.

It is based on a major scientific discovery, the "Integral System", by Professor Petros (Australia) and Professor Ulmsten (Sweden) who proposed that bowel and bladder problems originate mainly from a damaged vagina or the ligaments which support it and not from the organs themselves. One application, the midurethral sling operation, also invented by Petros & Ulmsten, has changed the lives of millions of women since the year 2000, converting a painful operation involving a 12 day hospital stay with indwelling urinary catheters, to a fairly painless day-care operation.

The experience of myself and other surgeons confirms cure or major improvement of other symptoms, urgency, nocturia, pelvic pain and bowel incontinence, following similar day-care repair of other ligaments.

It takes many years for such a radical change in thinking to become widely known. This book is timely. It informs women how damaged vaginal ligaments can cause specific problem and how such problems can be cured or improved with a time-efficient pelvic floor regime, or with minimally invasive surgery.

前言——本书的特色

Bernhard Liedl 医生，国际盆底外科联盟主席，慕尼黑，德国

本书是基于澳大利亚 Petros 教授和瑞典 Ulmsten 教授关于"整体理论"的重大科学发现，即肠道和膀胱发生的问题主要源于阴道或支持阴道的韧带受损，而不是器官本身。其中，尿道中段悬吊术（midurethral sling）的应用也源自 Petros 教授和 Ulmsten 教授的这一理论，它将需要住院 12 天且留置尿管的痛苦手术转变成近似无痛的日间手术。自 2000 年开始，该术式改善了数百万女性的生活。

本人和其他医生的相关经历也表明，经日间手术修复韧带后，尿急、夜尿、盆腔疼痛和粪失禁等症状可得到治愈或显著改善。

这种思维上的根本转变需要很多年才能广为人知。本书的出版非常及时。它将告诉女性，阴道韧带损伤是如何导致特定的临床疾病，以及如何通过及时有效的盆底系统管理或者微创手术来治愈或改善这些疾病。

In this 2nd Edition, Dr Darren Gold has added a valuable chapter on the colorectal manifestations of loose ligaments, constipation, fecal incontinence, haemorrhoids, anal fissures and other bowel conditions. Liedl B Abteilung für Urogenitale Chirurgie und Urologie, Beckenbodenzentrum München, Denningerstrasse 44, D − 81679 München, Germany President International Collaboration of Pelvic Floor Surgeons President International Society for Pelviperineology

The Key Messages of the Book

Though symptoms seem to come from the bladder and bowel, the actual cause is looseness in the ligaments which support them. Using actual patient stories, we show how a wide variety of symptoms and prolapse can be improved or cured by strengthening the damaged ligaments either with day-care surgery, or in less severe cases, simple pelvic floor exercises.

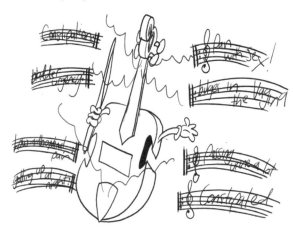

Fig1　The Pelvic floor Orchestra

在本版次(第 2 版)中,Darren Gold 医生增加了一个非常有价值的章节,就是韧带松弛引起的结直肠相关临床表现,如便秘、粪失禁、痔疮、肛裂和其他肠道症状。

本书的精髓

虽然很多症状似乎来源于膀胱和肠道,但真正的病因是其支持韧带的松弛。我们通过真实的病例,展示了各种不同的脱垂相关症状是如何通过加强受损韧带的日间手术得以改善或治愈,以及轻症患者甚至仅通过盆底训练即可得到改善。

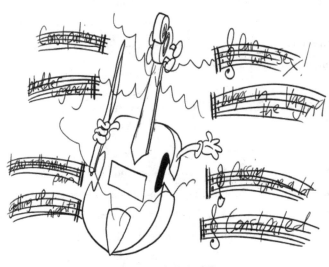

图 1　盆底管弦乐队

Think of the pelvis as an orchestra. The different ligaments, muscles and nerves of the pelvic floor work in harmony like the instruments of an orchestra. Each contributes differently to the final sound. When all the instruments are in tune, the music flows. If an instrument is broken, the music is out of tune. And so it is with the pelvic floor. Any damaged structure may cause problems. Damaged ligaments cause most of the problems, because so many structures depend on them for normal function. As each instrument has its own sound, so each ligament has a different symptom when things go wrong. The symptoms are represented by wrong notes, constipation, bladder urgency, low abdominal pain, getting up at night to pass urine, pain or urine loss with intercourse, constipation, bulges in the vagina, pain in the vagina or lower abdomen and passing urine frequently.

How this book is structured—holistically, like an orchestra

A conventional book lists symptoms and provides long lists of explanations and treatments. This book looks at the pelvis holistically. Think of the pelvis as an orchestra. The bladder, bowel and uterus represent musical instruments. The brain is the conductor and it co-ordinates the instruments to produce a harmonious sound. In the same way that strings are essential to the function of the instruments, ligaments are essential to the function of say, the uterus. Just as a loose string can distort the sound emitting from the instrument and indeed, the orchestra, so can a loose ligament cause prolapse of the uterus and multiple apparently unrelated symptoms.

　　我们将盆底比喻成一个管弦乐队。盆底不同的韧带、肌肉和神经就像管弦乐队的各种乐器一样协同演奏。每种乐器都对最终的声音有着不同的贡献。当所有的乐器都合拍时，音乐就会流畅。当一个乐器出现故障时，音乐就会走调。盆底也是如此，任何一个结构受损都可能会引发临床症状，大部分问题都是受损的韧带引起的。因为许多结构都依赖韧带才能发挥正常的功能。就像每个乐器都有自己的音色一样，每条韧带受损时都会带来不同的症状。错误的音符代表了这些症状，如便秘、尿急、下腹疼痛、夜尿、性交痛或性交时漏尿、便秘、阴道块物脱出、阴道或下腹部疼痛以及尿频等。

本书的架构——整体性，就像一个管弦乐队

　　传统书本会列举症状，并给出长长的解释和治疗方法。但本书不同，它将盆底想象成一个管弦乐队，从整体上对盆底进行研究。膀胱、肠管和子宫就像各种不同的乐器，大脑是指挥官，它协调各种乐器发出和谐的声音。就像琴弦对乐器的功能至关重要一样，韧带对子宫的作用也是如此。正如一根松掉的琴弦会扭曲乐器和整个管弦乐队发出的声音，松弛的韧带也会导致子宫脱垂和多种看似不相关的症状。

Like the instruments of an orchestra, the ligaments are grouped as front, middle and back. Each group of ligaments has its own specific symptoms and prolapses, exemplified in a series of typical patient histories in chapters 4, 5 & 6. A simple treatment philosophy follows: fix the ligaments and you cure the symptoms and the prolapse. We proceed to explain why, for example, loose front ligaments may cause stress incontinence (urine loss on coughing), why loose middle ligaments may cause cystocele (bladder prolapse) & chronic urinary infections or why loose back ligaments may cause dragging pain, urgency ("can't hold on") and nocturia (getting up at night to pass urine). Because diagrams are essential to this understanding, we recommend they be studied carefully, so readers obtain sufficient knowledge to meaningfully discuss their specific problem with their doctor.

A Short History of Incontinence

Since the beginning of time, incontinence has been accepted as part of ageing. Women didn't talk about it. Doctors never asked about it. Women, many of tender age, suffered, a passive conspiracy of silence. The general thinking behind pelvic floor problems has not altered in 100 years. It is symptom based. If a patient cannot "hold on" (urgency) goes to the toilet frequently during the day (frequency) or gets up at night to pass urine (nocturia) her bladder is said to be "unstable" and not curable. It is treated with marginally effective drugs, a multibillion dollar, highly marketed industry. Nor is any cure considered possible for some types of chronic pelvic pain and leakage of faeces. The only condition considered surgically curable has been stress incontinence (urine leakage on coughing).

像管弦乐队的乐器一样，韧带分为前部、中部和后部。每组（受损的）韧带都有其特定的症状和脱垂表现，在第四、第五和第六章会列举一系列典型的病例。一个简单的治疗理念是：修复韧带就能治愈脱垂和相关症状。关于这一理念，我们将在各章节做进一步解释。例如，为什么前部韧带的松弛会导致压力性尿失禁（咳嗽时漏尿），为什么中部韧带的松弛会导致膀胱膨出（膀胱脱垂）和慢性尿路感染，为什么后部韧带的松弛会导致牵拉痛、尿急（忍不住尿）和夜尿（晚上起床排尿）。因为图表是理解的基础，因此我们建议读者仔细研究示意图以获得足够的知识，从而能更有效地与医生讨论自己的具体问题。

尿失禁的简短历史

最初，尿失禁被认为是衰老的一种表现，女性从不讨论它，医生也从不提及它。然而，许多年轻女性也承受着被动的"缄默密约"之苦。对盆底疾病的总体认知 100 年来都没有什么改变，盆底疾病是基于症状的，如果患者不能"憋住"（尿急）、白天频繁上厕所（尿频）或晚上多次起来小便（夜尿），那她可能是因为有一个"不稳定的"膀胱，而这类疾病是无法治愈的。在临床治疗中，往往只能应用一些疗效不佳的药物，而这是一个价值数十亿美元、高度市场化的产业。对于某些类型的慢性盆腔疼痛和粪失禁而言，几乎没有任何治愈的可能。唯一可以手术治愈的症状是压力性尿失禁（咳嗽时漏尿）。

Our Aims

One aim in writing this book is to acquaint women with a revolution in thinking, that the source of most of these symptoms is damage to the vaginal ligaments, not the actual organ. We use a scientifically tested method to treat the above conditions. It is called the Integral System and it works by strengthening the vaginal ligaments with special exercises, or with new "keyhole" surgery methods.

A second more important aim is to empower women with sufficient knowledge to more meaningfully discuss their problems with their physician. We explain how the bladder and bowel work, why they don't and how they can be treated. This method is not confined to incontinence and prolapse. This is what a 34 year old patient said after her pelvic pain was cured.

"I was almost suicidal after interminable attacks of pain on my right side. It has now been a week since the operation and I feel like a rabbit that has been released from a trap. My mind keeps scanning up and down my body searching for the pain which for so long has been my centre and focus. "

It is not that this method is experimental. The midurethral sling (or TVT) has already revolutionized the treatment of urinary stress incontinence for millions of women. Not quite so well known is that repair of loose ligaments in the back part of the vagina may cure nocturia, frequency, urgency, not emptying properly and dragging low abdominal pain. A series of personal histories from patients brings further insights to a reader with similar problems. In keeping with our theme, "A Conspiracy of Silence", the deep emotional disturbance, which often accompanies these conditions, is highlighted.

我们的目标

撰写本书的目的之一，是让女性的思想认识发生革命性转变，即这些症状的根源是阴道韧带的损伤，而不是器官本身的病变。我们使用一种经过科学检验的方法来治疗上述情况。它被称为"整体理论系统"，即通过特殊的训练或新的"锁孔"小切口手术来加强阴道韧带。

第二个更重要的目的，是使女性获得足够的知识，以便与医生更有意义地讨论她们的问题。我们将解释膀胱和肠管是如何工作的，为什么它们会出现问题，以及如何治愈这些问题。这种疗法不局限于尿失禁和脱垂。以下是一位 34 岁的患者在盆腔疼痛治愈后所说的话。

"无休止的右侧腹痛，几乎让我想要自杀。现在手术已过去一周，我感觉自己就像是一只冲出牢笼的兔子，潜意识里仍上下搜寻那个长期以来占据我生活重心的痛点，但它消失了！"

这并不是试验性的方法。尿道中段吊带（或 TVT）是已经彻底改变了数百万压力性尿失禁女性的治疗方法。不过鲜为人知的是，修补阴道后部松弛的韧带可以用于治疗夜尿、尿频、尿急、排便不尽和下腹坠痛等。本书中一系列患者的个人经历能够帮助有类似问题的读者理解得更加深刻。为了与我们的主题"缄默的密约"保持一致，我们在书中尤其强调了与盆底症状伴生的极度情感困扰。

（广州医科大学附属第一医院妇产科，梁雪早 译，张晓薇 校）

The History of the Kvinno Centre (Perth, Australia) 1991 – 2009

by Professor Peter Petros

A snapshot of pelvic floor medicine before 1991

In 1991, treatment of incontinence mainly followed the International Continence Society's (ICS) recommendations. These recommendations were based on Urodynamics, which measured bladder pressure. If the pressure rose to a certain level, a diagnosis of "unstable bladder" was made. Treatment with drugs was recommended. However, most women ceased drug treatment because of side effects. Many women, who could not hold on (urgency), with no evidence of an "unstable bladder" on Urodynamic testing were sent to psychologists and psychiatrists. The reason? The problem must have been "psychological" (in their head), because these bladder tests were deemed to be objective and therefore, infallible.

Surgery for incontinence was only recommended when there was no "unstable bladder". In any case, surgery was painful, with large abdominal incisions, 10 to 14 days in hospital, inability to pass urine and long periods with catheters in the bladder. Surgery for prolapse had not altered for 100 years. Symptoms such as getting up at night to pass urine (nocturia), inability to hold on (urgency), going to the toilet frequently (frequency), chronic pelvic pain were all deemed incurable and treated with mainly ineffective drugs.

Kvinno 中心简介（澳大利亚，珀斯）
1991—2009

Peter Petros 教授　著

1991年前的盆底医学概况

1991年前，尿失禁的治疗主要遵循国际尿控协会（International Continence Society，ICS）的建议。这些建议是基于测量膀胱压的尿动力学。如果压力上升到一定程度，即可诊断为"不稳定性膀胱"，推荐使用药物治疗。但是，由于不良反应太大，多数妇女最终停止药物治疗。而那些尿动力学检查未提示"不稳定性膀胱"的妇女，则被转诊到心理学家和精神科医生那里。原因是什么？因为临床医生认为，膀胱测压是客观的，因此是绝对可靠的。如果尿动力学检查正常还出现盆底问题，那一定是"心理"上的问题（头脑问题）。

没有"不稳定性膀胱"的尿失禁患者才被推荐进行手术治疗。手术会有很大的腹部切口，需住院 10～14 天，由于排尿困难要长时间留置导管，这对任何患者都是痛苦的。治疗脱垂的手术则在近 100 年都没有什么改变。诸如起夜小便（夜尿）、无法憋尿（急迫）、频繁上厕所（尿频）、慢性盆腔疼痛等症状，都被认为是无法治愈的，主要治疗手段往往是基本无效的药物治疗。

The Kvinno Centre was a private clinic, the first clinic in the world based on the Integral System method. It was the source of the science and the histories in this book. Established in 1991 on the South Bank of the Swan River in Perth, Western Australia, it evolved from the original scientific work carried out by myself and John Papadimitriou, Professor of Pathology at the Royal Perth Hospital, Western Australia in 1987. We discovered a method for creating artificial ligaments to reinforce damaged ligaments in the pelvic region. This technique was applied to the first midurethral sling operations performed between 1988 and 1989. These operations were successful in curing both stress and urge incontinence, required only a day stay in hospital and led to the Integral System method.

In 1990, Professor Ulf Ulmsten, a prominent Professor from the University of Uppsala, Sweden, visited Royal Perth Hospital to review the patients and the results of the original operations. A rich scientific collaboration between Professor Ulmsten and myself followed for some years, producing the revolutionary TVT day-care operation for cure of urinary stress incontinence (urine loss on coughing). By 1995, the Integral System was delivering significant cure rates for many of the symptoms not previously considered curable by the majority of specialists in the field.

All this produced a classic conflict situation, as summarized by the Austrian philosopher Schopenhauer.

All truth passes through three stages. First, it is ridiculed. Second, it is violently opposed. Third, it is accepted as being self-evident.

Kvinno 中心是一家私人诊所，也是世界上第一家基于"整体理论系统"疗法的诊所。它也是本书中相关理论和治疗故事的来源。它成立于 1991 年，位于西澳大利亚珀斯（Perth）的天鹅河南岸（the South Bank of the Swan River）。由我和西澳大利亚皇家珀斯医院（the Royal Perth Hospital，Western Australia）的病理学教授 John Papadimitriou 1987 年的前期科研工作发展而来。我们发现了一种形成人工韧带以加固盆腔区域受损韧带的疗法。该技术在 1988—1989 年用于世界首例尿道中段悬吊术。这种仅需住院 1 天就能成功治愈压力性尿失禁和急迫性尿失禁的术式，最终形成了"整体理论系统"疗法。

1990 年，瑞典乌普萨拉大学（University of Uppsala）的著名教授 Ulf Ulmsten 访问了皇家珀斯医院（Royal Perth Hospital），看望了术后患者，评估了最初手术的结果。Ulmsten 教授和我本人之间的亲密科学合作持续了多年，并最终创造了革命性的 TVT 日间手术治疗压力性尿失禁（咳嗽时漏尿）。截至 1995 年，"整体理论系统"为那些曾经被该领域大多数专家认为无法治愈的病症提供了很高的治愈率。

正如奥地利哲学家叔本华（Schopenhauer）总结的那样，所有这些都表现为一种典型的冲突局面。

所有的真理都经历 3 个阶段：首先被嘲笑，然后被强烈反对，最后被理所当然地接受。

In spite of this marginalization, rapid progress occurred. In the intervening years, 1991 to 2009, the Centre became a reference point of last resort for women of all ages who were told no cure was available for their conditions. Many of their stories are highlighted later in this book. Many interstate and international surgeons visited Perth to observe the patients, the method and the operations. More ground-breaking scientific papers evolved in those years.

By 2009, the TVT operation for cure of urinary stress incontinence had become the world-wide standard for this condition. Former critics embraced it and promoted themselves as leaders in the field. The more controversial parts of the Integral System, such as surgical cure of unstable bladder symptoms and chronic pelvic pain have progressed more slowly and have still to achieve universal acceptance.

By 2009, heavy academic demands internationally created a conflict for me, whether to continue my work in the clinic in Perth or to accept the many invitations from Europe, Asia, North and South America to travel and teach the wider aspects of the Integral System and its surgical operations. After 18 years the clinic closed. By then, my textbook, "The Female Pelvic Floor," by PEP Petros, Springer Heidelberg, had become widespread, with translations into 8 languages, including Spanish, German, Chinese, Japanese.

Although the original Kvinno Centre is no longer operating in Perth, my work in teaching the Integral System continues internationally, with many thousands of physicians worldwide following its teachings in all or in part.

尽管遭遇了排斥，但"整体理论系统"的发展仍十分迅速。从 1991 年到 2009 年，Kvinno 中心成为那些被告知无法治愈的所有年龄段女性的最后依赖。她们的许多故事在本书后续的内容中都有所展现。许多国内外的医生来珀斯观摩，学习治疗方法和手术过程。在那些年里，更多具有开拓性的科学论文不断涌现。

到 2009 年，TVT 手术治疗压力性尿失禁已经成为世界范围内的标准术式。曾经的批评人士也接受了它，并成为该领域的领导者。但"整体理论系统"中比较有争议的部分，如外科手术治疗不稳定性膀胱症状及慢性盆腔疼痛的进展较慢，仍有待全世界的认可。

2009 年，国际上对学术的强烈需求使我内心矛盾，是继续在珀斯的诊所工作，还是接受来自欧洲、亚洲、北美和南美洲的邀请，开启行程去广泛传授"整体理论"及其手术技术？ Kvinno 诊所运营了 18 年，彼时，我的著作《女性骨盆底》[PEP Petros 著，由斯普林格出版社（海德堡）出版发行]，已被翻译成包括西班牙语、德语、中文、日语在内的 8 种语言，广为传播。

尽管在珀斯，最初的 Kvinno 中心早已不再运行，但我对"整体理论系统"的教学工作在国际上不断推进，数以千计的医生在全部或部分地遵循它的理念。

We have applied the 'Integral System' over the past 10 years at the Kvinno Center , Hannover, to patients from all parts of Germany. We confirm outstanding results for non-surgical and surgical treatments for stress incontinence , prolapse and symptoms such as urgency , nocturia , pelvic pain , bowel and bladder incontinence.

Dr Med. Bettina Rushmeier MD, Professor
Dr Med Klaus Goeschen MD PhD,
Kvinno Center, Hannover Germany.

在过去的 10 年里，我们在汉诺威的 Kvinno 中心，运用"整体理论系统"治疗来自于德国各地的患者。我们确信非手术和手术治疗对于压力性尿失禁、脱垂以及诸如尿急、夜尿、盆腔疼痛、粪失禁的症状疗效显著。

Bettina Rushmeier 医生, 医学博士, 教授

Klaus Goeschen 医生, 医学博士, 哲学博士

德国, 汉诺威, Kvinno 中心

（上海交通大学医学院附属第六人民医院妇产科，陈立奇 译，吴氢凯 校）

Overview

In the first chapter, the reader is introduced to the bladder, uterus and rectum and how they function.

Chapter 2 explains how problems arise in these organs because of damage to the vagina or its ligaments.

Chapter 3 gives a brief summary of treatment options.

In keeping with our theme of ligament damage, chapters 4, 5 & 6 describe typical patient stories and the specific symptoms and prolapses associated with the front, middle and back ligaments, with which the reader may be able to identify.

In Chapter 7, Dr Darren Gold, Colorectal and Pelvic Floor Reconstructive Surgeon, gives a brief outline of how these same ligaments can cause haemorrhoids, chronic constipation, fecal incontinence, anal fissures etc. with illustrative case histories.

Chapter 8 Discusses general care, nutrition and fluid management

In Chapter 9, a typical visit to a clinic is described. A patient gives her history of what is involved in visiting such a clinic, the tests and treatments typically offered, the consent process, the surgery and the after surgery period.

This is followed by Chapter 10, a short summary and conclusion.

Peter Petros
Joan McCredie
Patricia Skilling

概述

第一章,介绍膀胱、子宫、直肠以及其功能。

第二章,阐述阴道或其韧带的损伤如何导致这些器官的疾病。

第三章,简述治疗方案的选择。

为了与我们的主题——韧带损伤相一致,第四～六章描述了一些典型患者的故事,以及与前部、中部、后部韧带相关的具体症状和脱垂类型,方便读者识别。

第七章,结直肠和盆底重建外科医生 Darren Gold 用典型病例,概述了这些相同的韧带是如何引起痔疮、慢性便秘、粪失禁以及肛裂等问题的。

第八章,讨论综合护理、营养及液体管理。

第九章,描述一次典型的诊所就诊经历。一位患者描述了她在这家诊所的就诊过程,包括常用检查和治疗,知情同意的流程,手术以及术后康复。

第十章,简要的总结和结论。

彼得·佩特洛斯
琼·麦克格蕾迪
帕特里夏·斯奇琳

(上海交通大学医学院附属第六人民医院妇产科,徐玮 译,吴氢凯 校)

Contents

目　录

CHAPTER 1　Causation of Incontinence and Prolapse

This diagram shows how the babyrs head severely stretches the vagina and its ligaments to cause looseness which is the main cause of bladder and bowel prolapse, incontinence and pelvic pain.

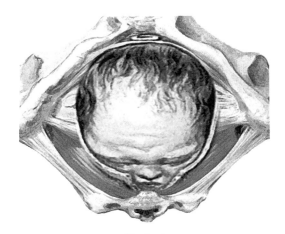

Fig 1 – 1

How do I know if I have a problem?

If you answer yes to one of the following, you have a problem.
1. You lose urine during exertion or coughing. This is called stress incontinence.

第一章　失禁和脱垂的病因

图 1-1 显示了分娩过程中婴儿的头部是如何极度拉伸阴道及其韧带,导致其松弛。韧带肌肉的松弛是膀胱和肠道脱垂、各种失禁和盆腔疼痛的主要原因。

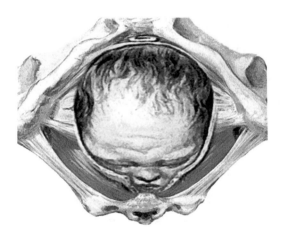

图 1-1　分娩

我如何知道自己的盆底出现了问题?

如果您对下列任何一个问题的回答是肯定的,那么您的盆底就有问题了。

1. 您在用力或咳嗽时出现漏尿,这被称为压力性尿失禁(stress incontinence)。

2. You can't "hold on". This is called urge incontinence.
3. You can't empty your bladder properly.
4. You have bowel soiling. This is called faecal incontinence.
5. You feel a lump in your vagina. This is called prolapse.
6. You have dragging lower abdominal or pelvic pain.

How serious is my problem?

Assessment by the patient. This question "how serious in my problem" is not so easy to answer, as symptoms vary and patients' perceptions vary. A simple rule is to seek help if it is interfering with your quality of life. If the problem is mild and not bothersome, no action is required.

Assessment by the clinic. The doctor has a different perspective: a) to assess which ligaments have been damaged and b) to assess the seriousness of the problem. An accurate assessment is paramount. The doctor uses various tests to decide which treatment to recommend. Later in the book, we devote a chapter to this subject, 'A Typical Visit to the Clinic', the experience of one patient as she goes through the whole process: assessment, consent and decision for treatment.

Understanding Your Vagina, Bladder, Bowel, and How They Should Work

"Looseness in the vaginal ligaments is the ultimate cause of prolapse, bladder and bowel symptoms and some types of pelvic pain" -**Integral System.**

2. 您不能憋尿,这被称为急迫性尿失禁(urge incontinence)。

3. 您不能正常排空膀胱。

4. 您有把大便拉在裤子里的经历,这被称为粪失禁(faecal incontinence)。

5. 您感到阴道里有块物脱出,这称为脱垂(prolapse)。

6. 您有牵扯样下腹痛或盆腔疼痛。

我的问题有多严重?

患者自我评估:"我的问题有多严重"这个问题并不容易回答,因为不同患者的症状不同,其感知能力也存在差异。一个简单的原则是,如果您的生活质量受到了影响,那就需要寻求帮助。如果问题轻微而且不影响生活,则不需要采取任何措施。

医生评估:医生有不同的视角。①定位评估:评估哪些韧带受损。②定性评估:评估疾病的严重程度。准确的评估至关重要。医生应用各种检查来决定应该推荐哪种治疗方案。本书中,我们用"一次典型的就诊经历"这样一个章节来描述这个主题。该章节叙述了一名患者经历的"评估、知情同意和接受治疗"的整个就诊过程。

了解您的阴道、膀胱、肠道,以及它们的工作机制

"盆腔韧带松弛是导致脱垂、膀胱和肠道症状以及某些类型盆腔疼痛的根本原因"——**整体理论系统**

Symptoms

A symptom is a warning bell from the brain that something is wrong with some part of the body. As regards the bladder and bowel, there are 2 types of symptoms, inability to retain the urine or faeces, "incontinence", or inability to empty. A third related symptom is dragging pelvic pain.

Prolapse

A prolapse is a bulge or lump in the vagina. A bulge in the fornt wall of the vagina is called a cystocoele. A bulge in the back wall of the vagina is called a rectocoele. Descent of the uterus into the up-per part of the vagina is called "uterine prolapse". Symptoms may occur with large or even minimal prolapse.

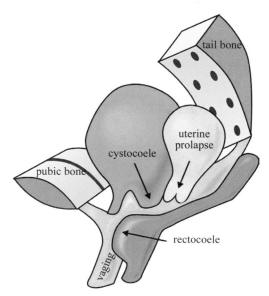

Fig 1 – 2 The different types of prolapses

症状

症状是大脑发出的警告信号,表明身体的某些部位出现了问题。至于膀胱和直肠的问题,通常有两类症状:一种是不能储存尿液或粪便(失禁),另一种是不能排空。第三种相关症状是迁延不愈的盆腔疼痛。

脱垂

脱垂(prolapse)表现为阴道内有组织物膨出或形成块物。阴道前壁的膨出称为膀胱膨出(cystocele);阴道后壁的膨出称为直肠膨出(rectocele)。子宫下降至阴道上段以下称为子宫脱垂(uterine prolapse)。严重的脏器脱垂甚至只是轻微的脱垂均有可能导致不适症状。如图 1 - 2 所示。

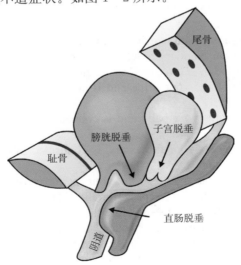

图 1 - 2　各种脏器的脱垂

The bladder, uterus and bowel push into the vagina as a lump because the structures (ligaments) which suspend them are weakened. See Fig1 – 3 for perspective.

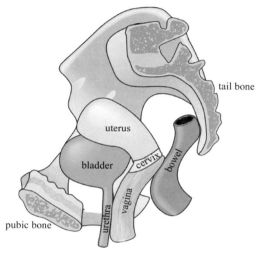

Fig1 – 3   Bladder, Vagina, Uterus, Bowel and their outlet tubes.

Side view organs positioned in a standing body.

This is what your bladder, bowel and uterus look like viewed from the side, Fig 1 – 3. Think of these organs as storage containers.

The bladder stores your urine and is connected to the outside by a tube, the urethra.

The uterus stores your baby and is connected to the outside by a tube, the vagina.

The rectum stores your faeces and is connected to the outside by a tube called the anus.

Your baby and the blood from your periods pass through the vagina. Urine and faeces pass through the urethra and anus. Muscles compress these tubes to close them and stretch them open for emptying. The bone in front of your bladder is called the pubic bone and the bone behind your rectum is called the sacrum or tail bone.

The vagina supports the bladder above and the rectum (bowel) below, so anything which damages the vagina or the ligaments

因为器官的支持结构（韧带）松弛、薄弱，膀胱、子宫和直肠突入阴道内形成块物。如图1-3所示。

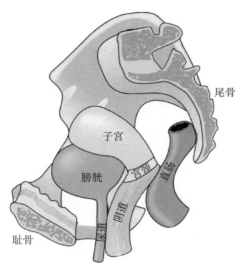

图1-3　膀胱、阴道、子宫、直肠及其出口

站立位的器官位置（侧面观）。

这就是从侧面看膀胱、直肠和子宫的形态，可以把这些器官比作储存的容器（见图1-3）。

膀胱（bladder）：储存尿液并通过尿道与外界相通。

子宫（uterus）：是孕育胎儿的地方，并通过阴道与外界相通。

直肠（rectum）：储存大便，通过肛门与外界相通。

胎儿和月经血通过阴道排出体外，尿液和粪便通过尿道和肛门排出体外。各通道通过周围肌肉收缩时关闭、舒张时开放来控制排泄。膀胱前方的骨头称为耻骨，直肠后方的骨头称为骶骨或尾骨。

阴道（vagina）：支撑着前上方的膀胱和后下方的直肠，所以

which support it can also affect the bladder and rectum.

The uterus is a very important structure. Note how the ligaments and both walls of the vagina attach to the uterus. The lower part of the uterus is called the cervix and it is situated right at the back of your vagina. The cervix is where your Pap smear is taken from.

The perineal body (PB) is a firm structure which separates the lower part of the vagina from the back passage. It supports the vagina from below. If this is damaged, the rectum (bowel) may bulge forwards into the vagina. This is called a rectocele.

A ligament is like a thick cord. Ligaments suspend the vagina and uterus from above, exactly like a suspension bridge, Fig 1 − 4.

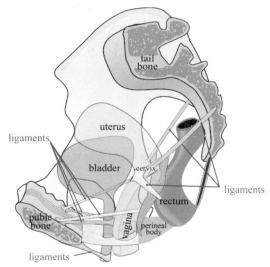

Fig 1 − 4   The ligaments suspend the organs from above like a suspension bridge. The perineal body (PB) supports the vagina from below and separates the vagina from the rectum.

The uterus acts like the keystone of an arch and so it has a critically important role in supporting the vagina, bladder and bowel. Its removal may predispose to prolapse, bladder, bowel and pain symptoms whose onset may be delayed until after the menopause.

阴道的肌肉或其韧带的损伤也可能影响到膀胱和直肠的功能。

子宫(the uterus)：是非常重要的结构,需注意子宫周围的韧带和阴道前后壁是如何与子宫相连的。子宫的下部称为宫颈,其刚好位于阴道的顶端,宫颈也是集取细胞进行涂片检查的部位。

会阴体(the perineal body, PB)：是位于阴道下段和肛管之间的一层坚韧的组织结构,从下方支撑着阴道结构。如果会阴体结构受损,直肠可能会向前、向下膨出至阴道内,这称为直肠膨出(rectocele)。

韧带(ligament)：如同粗的绳索,就像吊桥一样,从上方悬吊着子宫和阴道,如图1-4所示。

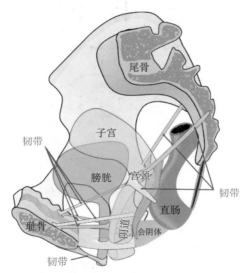

图1-4　像吊桥一样,韧带从上方悬吊着器官。会阴体位于阴道和直肠之间,其从下方支撑阴道

子宫的作用就像拱门的拱心石,在维持阴道、膀胱和直肠的正常解剖位置中发挥了关键作用。切除子宫后可能更易发生脱垂、膀胱/直肠不适和盆腔疼痛,而这些疾病一般都在绝经后才出现,如图1-5所示。

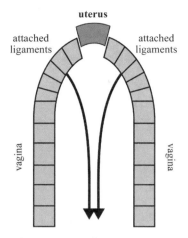

Fig 1 – 5   **The uterus acts like the keystone of an arch**

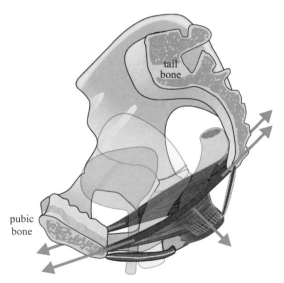

Fig 1 – 6   The pelvic muscles (dark red) wrap around and support the vagina (blue), bladder (green), and bowel (brown) from below. Forward contraction (arrows) closes the urethra and anus; backward contraction (arrows) opens the urethra and anus.

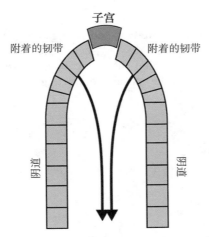

图 1-5 子宫的作用就像拱门的拱心石一样

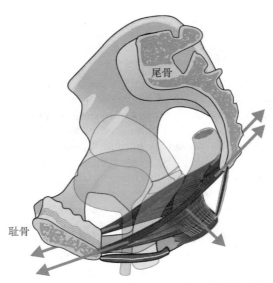

图 1-6 盆腔肌肉(暗红色)包绕阴道(蓝色)、膀胱(绿色)、直肠(棕色),并从下方支撑着这些器官。这些肌肉向前收缩(箭头所示)可以使尿道和肛管闭合,向后收缩(箭头所示)则开放尿道和肛管

The red arrows indicate the directions where the muscles contract, backwards to open the urethral and anal tubes, forwards to close them. Some muscles are easy to feel. Place your fingers in the vagina and feel just behind the pubic bone. Push down hard or cough. You will feel the muscle contracting.

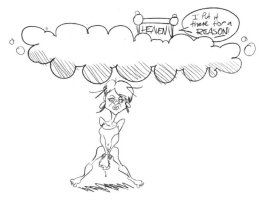

Fig 1 – 7

This is a confronting illustration. It shows a woman clutching her uterus which has come out of the vagina (prolapse). It emphasize the potentially catastrophic effects of hysterectomy (removal of the uterus). There is a modern culture of "Take the uterus out" on the basis that it has served its purpose. Many women adopt this viewpoint as they long to be free of their periods. Many doctors who deal with prolapse see the uterus as an obstacle to a proper repair of the prolapse and so they remove it. Yet, the uterus is a very important organ. It is the spiritual core of a woman, the place where she conceives and nurtures her babies. For many women it is the foundation stone of their femininity and some experience severe psychological reactions when it is removed. From a structural viewpoint, the uterus is very important, as it is the anchoring point for almost all the ligaments of the pelvis. Hysterectomy involves cutting these ligaments. In the longer term, this may cause prolapse, constipation, bladder and bowel incontinence. Our view is that the uterus is central to any ligament

14

红色箭头指示肌肉收缩的方向,向后收缩可开放尿道和肛管,向前收缩则关闭尿道和肛管。其中一些肌肉很容易被感觉到,比如将手指置入阴道内耻骨后方,然后增加腹压或者咳嗽,您会感觉到肌肉的收缩。

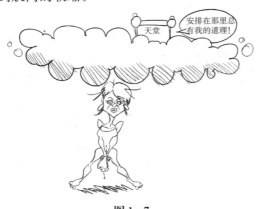

图 1-7

这是一张正面示意图,它描绘了一位女性紧握着从阴道掉出来的子宫(子宫脱垂),强调了切除子宫可能导致的灾难性影响。如今有种观点认为子宫的使命就是孕育生命,当子宫完成使命后就可以把它切除。许多女性采信了这种观点,因为她们渴望摆脱月经的烦恼。许多医生在治疗子宫脱垂时,也认为子宫是治愈这种疾病的障碍,因此要切除它。事实上,子宫是一个非常重要的器官,它是女性的精神支柱,是女性孕育胎儿的地方。对于许多女性而言,子宫是她们女性气质的基石。切除子宫后,一些女性会产生严重的心理反应。从结构上看,子宫是非常重要的,它是几乎所有盆腔韧带的锚定点,切除子宫就需要切断所有这些韧带。从长远来看,这可能导致脏器脱垂、便秘、尿失禁和粪失禁。我们的观点是,子宫是所有盆底韧带重建手术的关键,如果没有很好的理由,比如罹患严重的子宫出血或恶性

reconstruction and should not be removed without good reason, for example, heavy bleeding or cancer.

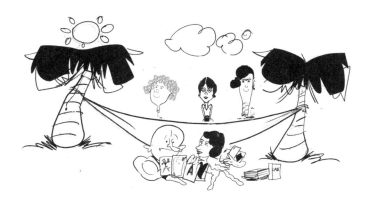

Fig 1 – 8   Everything normal, tight and in balance

The trees represent the pelvic skeleton. The vagina is attached to the skeleton by strong tight ligaments and everything is tensioned subconsciously by the pelvic muscles. In this situation, our little characters Betty Bladder, Andrea Anus, Ursula Uterus swing peacefully in the vaginal hammock which supports them. The brain has Lilli Ligament and Mickey Muscle on " automatic pilot", so they spend their time playing cards.

肿瘤等,就不应轻易切除它。

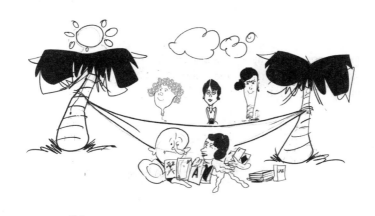

图 1-8　一切正常,松紧适宜,平衡相当

　　图 1-8 中的两棵树代表了盆腔的骨骼,阴道通过强有力的韧带附着于骨盆。盆底肌肉自主地维持着各个结构的张力。在这种情形下,我们的小主角们,膀胱贝蒂(Betty Bladder)、肛门安德莉亚(Andrea Anus)和子宫乌苏拉(Ursula Uterus)这些小姐们在阴道这个吊床上平静地摆荡着。大脑由韧带莉莉(Lilli Ligament)女士和肌肉米奇(Mickey Muscle)先生驾驭着,所以她们可以安心地玩纸牌了。

（中国医学科学院北京协和医院妇产科,田维杰 译,朱兰 校）

CHAPTER 2   How and Why Things
Go Wrong

The enormous amount of stretching which occurs at childbirth may damage the collagen of the vagina and its ligaments to cause prolapse and symptoms.

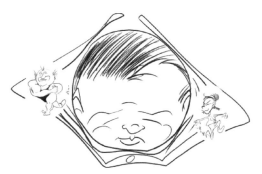

Fig 2 - 1   Causation: Mickey Muscle and Lilli
Ligament trapped, stretched, squeezed
and nowhere to go"

The head causes enormous stretching of the vagina and the ligaments as it descends. The diameter of a normal head is 9. 4 cm, while the pelvic diameter is only 12 - 13 cm. The adjoining structures, muscles and ligaments are necessarily compressed, torn or damaged.

Even when the head is at its smallest diameter, as in this picture, there is only 1. 5 cm on each side of the head where all the muscles and tissues must fit. The ligament and muscles are trapped, stretched, squeezed, sometimes crushed, with nowhere to go. It is a miracle that every woman's muscles and tissues are not destroyed. The reason for this is that a hormone from the

第二章　疾病发生、发展的原因及方式

经阴道分娩时,阴道的极度拉伸可损伤其胶原蛋白和韧带,导致脱垂及其相关症状。

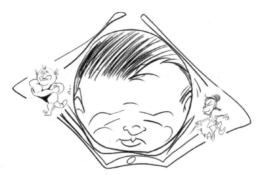

图 2 - 1　病因: 肌肉米奇(Mickey Muscle)先生和韧带莉莉(Lilli Ligament)女士被过度束缚、拉伸和挤压,它们无处可逃

随着胎头下降,阴道及其韧带受到极大的拉伸。正常胎头的直径为 9.4 cm,而骨盆直径仅为 12～13 cm。因此,当胎头通过阴道时,相邻的组织结构、肌肉和韧带均受到挤压、撕裂或损伤。

如图 2 - 1 所示,即使胎头以最小径线入盆,胎头的每一侧也仅有 1.5 cm 的间隙,所有的肌肉和组织都须与之相称。韧带和肌肉因无法移动,而被束缚、拉伸、挤压,甚至被撕裂。但奇妙的是,并非所有产妇的肌肉和组织都发生了损伤。究其原因,是

placenta loosens the bonds of the tissue molecules so they weaken and become elastic, making them far less vulnerable to tearing. Within 24 hours of the birth, this hormone disappears, the tissues rebound back to (almost) their normal state. In many women, however, the ligaments and vaginal wall remain stretched or torn and so they may develop bladder, bowel and pain symptoms. Others, whose tissues are excessively stretched or torn, may develop prolapse. Most develop prolapse and symptoms together. Even a minor prolapse may have major symptoms.

The two figures which follow graphically show the effect of overstretching on the top, front walls and back walls of the vagina, to cause prolapse and symptoms. These are detailed below.

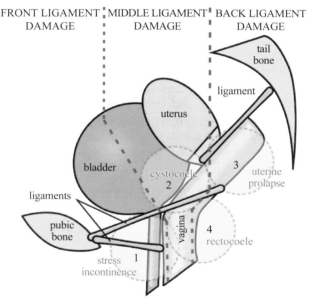

Fig 2 − 2 **Birthing damage side view shows how a head descending down the vagina may overstretch the vagina**

来自胎盘的激素使组织分子的结合变得松散，从而使肌肉变得更有弹性，也更不易被撕裂。这些激素在分娩后 24 小时内消失，组织（几乎）恢复到孕前的正常状态。但是，仍有许多女性的韧带和阴道壁处于拉伸或撕裂的状态，可能会出现膀胱、肠道和疼痛症状。如果组织被过度拉伸或撕裂，可能会发展成器官脱垂。多数情况下，脱垂和相应的症状都是同时出现的。轻微的脱垂也可伴随明显的症状。

图 2-2 和图 2-3 形象地描绘了过度拉伸对阴道顶部、前壁和后壁的影响，以及导致脱垂和相应症状的发生机制。详细说明如下：

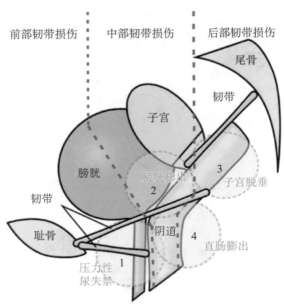

图 2-2 阴道分娩损伤侧视图，显示胎头沿阴道下降致阴道组织被过度拉伸

Front vaginal wall, front ligament damage: stress incontinence "1";
Front vaginal wall, middle ligament damage: cystocele "2".
Top of the vagina (apex): prolapse of uterus "3".
Back vaginal wall: rectocele "4".
Clarification Symptoms relate only to specific ligaments, front, middle and back.

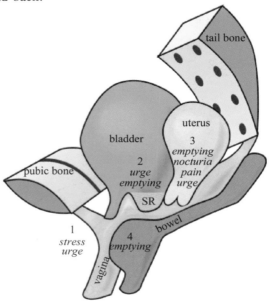

Fig 2 - 3   The various prolapses and symptoms which
may result from the damage caused in sites
1 - 4, Fig 2 - 2.

Damage to the front ligament of vagina '1' does not cause prolapse. The main problem is urine loss on coughing (stress incontinence) frequency and urgency.
Damage to the front wall of vagina, middle ligament damage '2' may cause protrusion of bladder into the vagina (cystocele). The stretch receptors nerves (SR) sense when the bladder is full. The main problems are difficulty in emptying the bladder, chronic bladder infections and urgency.

位点1.阴道前壁、前部韧带损伤：压力性尿失禁。

位点2.阴道前壁、中部韧带损伤：膀胱膨出。

位点3.阴道顶端（顶点）支持缺陷：子宫脱垂。

位点4.阴道后壁损伤：直肠膨出。

特别说明：症状与特定韧带（前、中、后部韧带）有关。

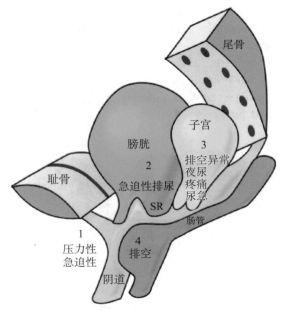

图2-3　各种器官脱垂和症状可能是图2-2所示位点1～4的损伤所致（SR：牵扯张感受器）

位点1.阴道前部韧带损伤：不会导致脱垂，主要导致咳嗽时不自主漏尿（压力性尿失禁）、尿频和尿急。

位点2.阴道前壁、中部韧带损伤：可导致膀胱突向阴道（膀胱膨出）。牵张感受器（stretch receptors，SR）可感知膀胱是否充盈。主要症状是膀胱排空困难、慢性膀胱炎和尿急。

23

Damage to the top of vagina ' 3 ' damages the back ligaments. This causes the uterus to fall down into the vagina (prolapse of the uterus). The main symptoms are chronic pelvic pain, getting up at night to pass urine (nocturia), difficulty in emptying the bladder, frequency and urgency.

Damage to back wall of vagina '4', the perineal body, may cause a protrusion of bowel into the vagina (rectocele). The main problem is difficulty in emptying the bowel. Sometimes a patient may need to press down with her finger in that area to facilitate opening her bowels.

Loose Ligaments Weaken the Muscles to Cause Symptoms and Prolapse. The pelvic muscles need a firm ligament attachment to work properly. Loose ligaments can lead to symptoms and prolapse.

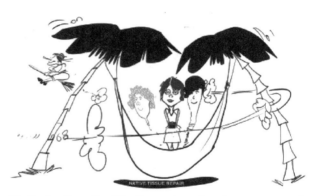

Fig 2 - 4 Causation The ligaments and vagina are too weak to contain the organs

位点 3.阴道顶部损伤：盆腔后部韧带损伤,会导致子宫落入阴道(子宫脱垂)。主要症状是慢性盆腔疼痛、夜间多次起床排尿(夜尿症)、排尿困难、尿频和尿急。

位点 4.阴道后壁和会阴体损伤：可能会导致直肠突向阴道(直肠膨出)。主要问题是排便困难,有时患者需要用手指按压该区域以协助排便。

韧带松弛使肌力减弱,引起脱垂和相应症状。肌肉需要牢固的韧带附着于骨盆才能正常工作,韧带松弛会导致相关症状和脱垂。

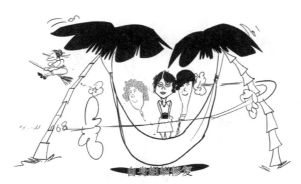

图 2-4 病因：韧带和阴道力量太弱,无法维持器官的正常位置

If the ropes are loose, the hammock (vagina) 'droops', so that Betty Bladder, Ursula Uterus and Andrea Anus bulge into the vagina. The woman perceives these as "lumps". It is clear from the diagram that just cutting out the bottom part of the lump (native tissue repair) will make things look better for a while, but it will not cure the problem. This is what standard vaginal repairs do. The ropes (ligaments) attaching the hammock to the tree remain elongated. To cure the problem, the ligaments have to be shortened and strengthened.

This is exactly what was done by the new TFS system which was used to cure the prolapses described in the patient stories.

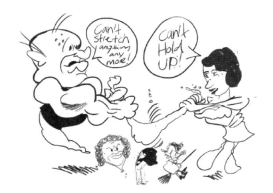

Fig 2 - 5   Causation 4 Everything stretched and out of balance

Lilli Ligament on one side says "Can't hold it up!"

Mickey Muscle on the other says "Can't stretch anything anymore!"

Once the ligaments are damaged, the vagina becomes loose, so the bladder, bowel and uterus fall down. Lilli Ligament can't hold up the vaginal hammock, so prolapses of the bladder (cystocele), uterus (uterine prolapse) and bowel (rectocele) may occur as lumps in the vagina. Nor can Mickey Muscle stretch the vagina, because the muscles need a firm ligament to contract against. So

如果绳索松弛,吊床(阴道)会"下垂",膀胱贝蒂、子宫乌苏拉和肛门安德莉亚会突向阴道,也就是女性感觉到的"块物"。从图2-4中可以清楚地看出,仅切除"块物"的底部组织(自身组织修复),可能在一段时间内看起来效果不错,不过没有解决根本问题,这就是常规的阴道修复手术。但这种手术后,把吊床连接到树上的绳索(韧带)仍处于拉伸状态。为了解决这个问题,必须缩短和加强韧带。

这正是新的组织固定系统(tissue fixation system,TFS)可用于治愈患者所描述脱垂症状的原理。

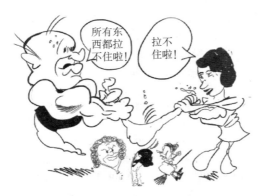

图2-5　病因: 组织过度拉伸,失去平衡

韧带莉莉在一侧说:"拉不住啦!"

肌肉米奇在另一侧说:"所有东西都拉不住啦!"

一旦韧带受损,阴道就会松弛,膀胱、肠管和子宫就会脱垂。韧带莉莉无法支撑阴道吊床,膀胱膨出、子宫脱垂和直肠膨出就会表现为阴道内块物。由于需要牢固的韧带来对抗肌肉收缩,韧带松弛使肌肉米奇无法伸展阴道,不能闭合尿道和肛门,从而导致尿失禁或粪失禁。最后,沿着韧带走行的神经也逐步失去支撑,不同类型的疼痛症状随之出现。

Mickey Muscle can no longer close the bladder or bowel tubes, so the woman loses urine or faeces. Finally, the nerves which run along the ligaments can no longer be supported, so several different types of pain can be experienced.

How loose ligaments cause symptoms

Incontinence is when urine and faeces leak out because the ligaments are overstretched and loose, so the muscles become floppy and cannot close the urethral or anal tubes.

Bladder and bowel emptying difficulties such as "dribbling, "can't empty", "constipation" are also caused by loose ligaments so that the muscles which open the urethra and anus also become floppy and cannot open properly.

Urinating frequently (frequency) and inability to hold on occurs when the special nerve endings in the bladder wall called stretch receptors (SR, Fig 2 − 3) fire off prematurely because the ligaments are too loose to support them. Stretch receptors give the brain a signal (urge feeling) that the bladder is full. If, for whatever reason, the vagina is loose, the "stretch receptors" fire off at a lower volume, so the patient goes more frequently during the day ("frequency") and during the night ("nocturia"). Because she cannot control the urge to empty, she reports it as "an uncontrollable desire to pass urine" ("urgency").

Pelvic Pain may be caused when the ligaments supporting the uterus are loose. These ligaments contain nerves. The prolapse may pull on these nerves to cause a "dragging pain".

Why Multiple Symptoms and Prolapses Occur at The Same Time It is evident from Fig 2 − 2 that a head descending down the vaginal canal is unlikely to damage just one single structure. That is why many problems occur together.

韧带松弛是如何导致相关症状发生的？

失禁：是指由于韧带被过度拉伸导致松弛，从而使肌肉松软，无法闭合尿道或肛门，最终导致尿液或粪便漏出。

膀胱和直肠排空困难：诸如"小便淋漓，无法排尽"、"便秘"等也由韧带松弛所致，韧带松弛引起肌力下降，无法正常开放尿道和肛门。

频繁排尿(尿频)和漏尿：发生于韧带过度松弛无法支撑阴道时，膀胱壁特殊神经末梢上的牵张感受器(stretch receptors, SR，见图2-3)提前发出冲动信号所致。牵张感受器向大脑发出膀胱充盈的信号(急迫感)。无论何种原因，只要出现阴道松弛，"牵张感受器"在膀胱容量较小时就会发出神经冲动，使患者无论在白天("尿频")还是在夜间("夜尿症")都会频繁地排尿。这种无法控制排尿的冲动，被描述为"无法控制的排尿欲望"("尿急")。

盆腔疼痛：可能源于支撑子宫的韧带发生松弛。这是因为这些韧带含有神经，脱垂会牵拉神经，从而导致"牵拉痛"。

为什么会同时出现多种症状和脱垂？ 从图2-2中可以很明显地看出，胎头向下通过阴道时，不可能仅损伤单一组织结构，因此许多问题可同时出现。

(北京大学人民医院妇产科，李松芳 译，王建六 校)

CHAPTER 3   A Brief Overview of Treatment Options

This section briefly discusses the main treatment options, both the traditional and the new.

Prevention 1. Does Caesarian section prevent prolapse and symptoms?

The short answer is only partly. The uterus has to prepare for labour. A hormone called "Relaxin" loosens the bonds which bind the collagen rods inside the ligaments and the vagina, so these stretch months before labour begins. This explains why pregnant women may develop bladder, bowel and pain symptoms well before labour starts. However, the process of labour creates even more stretching and more damage. Fortunately, most incontinence and pain symptoms which develop during pregnancy improve or disappear after delivery.

Prevention 2. Good bowel and urine habits

Nature always knows best. The system for bowel and bladder emptying is so highly developed we should listen to it. There is a simple rule for children and adults alike: "go when your bladder and bowel tell you to". This is especially so with the bowel. Injudicious straining when the faeces do not come can cause all sorts of problems. It is better to get up and go another time. If the problem is chronic, go onto a high bulk diet and seek advice from a physician.

第三章　治疗方案选择概述

本章简要讨论主要的传统疗法和新型疗法。

预防方法 1. 剖宫产能防止脱垂及其症状的发生吗？

下述简短答案只能在一定程度上回答这个问题。子宫必须为分娩做准备。孕期会释放一种叫做"松弛素"的激素，它会分解韧带和阴道组织内胶原蛋白间的连接，进而导致韧带的松弛。这些变化在分娩前数月就开始发生，这就解释了为什么孕妇在分娩前可能会出现膀胱、肠道的症状和疼痛。但是，分娩过程会产生更大的拉伸和损伤。幸运的是，妊娠期间出现的失禁及疼痛症状在分娩后大多会得到改善或消失。

预防方法 2. 养成良好的排便和排尿习惯

自然善知（nature always knows best）。人体肠道和膀胱排空系统已经进化得非常发达，我们应当遵循其自然规律。儿童和成人的原则都是一样的："当您的膀胱和肠道告诉您需要排空时，就该去排尿（便）了"。肠道系统尤其如此，在没有便意时用力屏大便是不明智的，往往会导致各种问题的产生，这种情况下最好的办法是站起身，等待有便意时再尝试。如果是慢性便秘，请加大饮食量并向医生寻求建议。

Prevention 3. Hormone Replacement Therapy ("HRT")

Major changes occur at the menopause. Ovaries cease to produce oestrogen, collagen breaks down, vaginal tissues weaken, prolapse and symptoms occur. Many patients experience hot flushes, some develop depression and many gain weight in different parts of the body. Logically, it seems reasonable to replace oestrogen. However, there are concerns, for example, increased susceptibility to breast cancer, (say from 4% to 5%), though this fear has not been fully substantiated. Vaginal oestrogens $2-3$ times per week are beneficial and are considered safe. Oestrogen HRT taken by mouth or applied to the skin on an ongoing basis may prevent osteoporosis and in some patients, depression. There is growing evidence that ovarian tumours originate from the Fallopian Tubes, so it is reasonable to remove only the tubes at hysterectomy and conserve the ovaries.

Vitamin D deficiency may affect the bones and perhaps the ligaments, as may testosterone. It is not generally known that testosterone is an extremely important hormone for women. Fifty per cent of testosterone is produced by the ovaries and is released directly into the bloodstream. Unlike the sudden drop in oestrogen production after the menopause, testosterone production falls slowly. Removal of the ovaries during hysterectomy does lead to sudden falls in testosterone levels. Common symptoms include impaired sexual desire, lessened wellbeing, loss of energy, depression and loss of bone. Colleagues working in specialist hormone clinics speak glowingly about the use of testosterone in menopausal women who have these symptoms. The area of hormone replacement is complex and controversial. Consultation with a physician specializing in hormone treatment is advised.

预防方法 3. 激素替代疗法

绝经期女性身体会发生重大变化。卵巢停止分泌雌激素，胶原蛋白分解，阴道组织逐渐变得薄弱、脱垂并出现相应症状。许多患者会出现潮热，一些人会出现抑郁症，还有许多人出现身体的不同部位发胖。从逻辑上讲，雌激素替代治疗似乎是合理的。然而，激素替代治疗仍有令人担忧的地方，例如：尽管未被完全证实，但有报道指出乳腺癌的易感性增加（从 4％增加到 5％）。每周 2～3 次在阴道内使用雌激素是有益处的，并且被认为是安全的。通过口服或皮贴连续使用雌激素替代治疗可以预防骨质疏松症，并可以预防一些患者抑郁症的发生。越来越多的证据表明，卵巢肿瘤起源于输卵管，因此在子宫切除术中仅切除输卵管并保留卵巢是合理的做法。

维生素 D 的缺乏可能会影响骨骼，甚至可能影响韧带，睾酮也可能有相似的作用。并不广为人知的是，睾酮对于女性而言是极其重要的激素。卵巢可产生 50％的睾酮，并直接释放到血液中。与绝经后雌激素分泌突然减少不同，睾酮分泌的降低相对缓慢。而子宫切除术中同时切除卵巢确实会导致睾酮水平的突然降低。常见症状包括：性欲减退，幸福感降低，精力不足，抑郁和骨量流失。激素专科门诊的医生们高度评价睾酮在具有这些症状的围绝经期妇女中的应用。激素替代治疗领域是复杂且有争议的。建议患者咨询专门从事激素治疗的医生。

Pessaries

Historically, sufficiently large rubber rings called vaginal pessaries have been inserted into the vagina to prevent the prolapse coming out of the vagina. This is the oldest treatment for prolapse, and it is still an option today, especially for women who are very ill or who wish to delay or avoid surgery. Pessary fitting is an art, as pessaries frequently fall out and may cause ulcers in the vagina with longterm usage. In our experience, pessaries are not welcome in the young sexually active woman.

Pessary usage is not confined to prolapse. In Germany, in patients with major symptoms but no significant prolapse, some physicians insert a 6 cm x 3 cm tampon-like cylinder with an attached string called "ProDry". This supports the bladder and the ligaments in the top part of the vagina, which can be quite effective in the short term, in improving urgency, nocturia and other symptoms. It is available on the net from Germany. Though it is essentially a large tampon, any use of the ProDry pessary should be under medical or nursing supervision. A similar effect, improvement in symptoms of urge, nocturia, pelvic pain can often be achieved by inserting a large menstrual tampon deep into the back part of the vagina, but only on a short term basis and only as a test, because long-term use of a tampon may absorb bacteria.

Though a pessary is still a useful option in the older patient, modern minimally invasive methods are increasingly consigning this method of treatment to history.

Drugs work by preventing the smooth muscle of the bladder from contracting. The problem is that they also work on other smooth muscles in the body to create side effects such as dry mouth, constipation, emptying difficulties to such an extent, that by 4 weeks, the vast majority of women cease taking their tablets.

子宫托

历史上,临床医生曾经把一个足够大的被称为"阴道子宫托"的橡胶圈放入阴道中,以防止脱垂的器官脱出阴道。这是最古老的治疗脱垂的方法,延用至今,特别适用于那些身体情况极差或希望推迟甚至避免手术的妇女。子宫托的放置是一门艺术,因为子宫托经常发生脱落,长期使用可能导致阴道溃疡。根据我们的经验,子宫托在性生活活跃的年轻女性中并不受欢迎。

子宫托的使用不限于脱垂。在德国,对一些症状严重但无显著脱垂的患者,有些医生在阴道内放置一个 6 cm×3 cm、附着有一根绳子的棉条状圆柱体,称为"ProDry"。它可以支撑膀胱和阴道顶部韧带,在短期内非常有效地改善尿急、夜尿症等其他症状。它可以在网上从德国购买。尽管 ProDry 子宫托本质上是一个大的卫生棉条,但它的任何使用均应在医疗或护理的监督下进行。通常,可以通过在阴道后部深处放入大的卫生棉条来达到类似的效果,从而改善尿急、夜尿、盆腔疼痛的症状,但是这只能在短期内使用,并且只能作为是否适用于"ProDry"的测试方法,因为长期使用卫生棉条可能会引起细菌感染。

尽管子宫托仍然是老年患者的有效选择,但现代微创手术治疗方法越来越让这种治疗方式成为历史。

药物治疗通过抑制膀胱平滑肌收缩而起作用。问题在于药物同样可以作用于身体的其他平滑肌,从而产生不良反应,例如口干、便秘、排空困难等,以至于治疗到 4 周时,绝大多数妇女都会停止服用。

Spinal nerve stimulation

This method requires considerable skill and knowledge. It is a treatment of last resort and is usually reserved for very severe cases of pelvic organ symptoms. Wires are inserted into the spinal nerves and an implanted battery sends impulses along the nerves. It is sometimes used for incontinence, but again, only as a last resort.

"Bladder Training" For Urgency Symptoms

The aim of "bladder training" is to train the brain to "hang on" for longer and longer periods. This transfers the symptom from "urge to go", to the pain of "hanging on", which is often beyond the patient's endurance.

Traditional Surgery for Cystocele or Rectocele

These methods "Native Tissue Repair", are more than 100 years old. The bulges in the vagina are simply cut out and the two edges sewn together. Damaged tissue is joined to damaged tissue. This explains why the cure rate for cystocele and rectocele repair is often poor. Furthermore, the vagina is a cylinder, so any removal of tissue will only narrow it or shorten it, potentially causing problems with sexual intercourse. We have seen a vagina reduced to the size of a thumb after 3 such operations. That is why most surgeons recommend that as little vagina as possible should be removed during these operations. If the ligaments are intact, these operations can work satisfactorily. Usually, however, the ligaments are also damaged. This explains the low rate of success of this type of excision surgery.

脊神经刺激

此方法需要掌握熟练的操作技能和扎实的理论知识。这是一种不得已而为之的治疗方法，通常适用于盆腔器官症状非常严重的情况。电极插入脊髓神经，置入的电池沿神经发送脉冲。有时可用于尿失禁，但需要再次强调，这种方法只能作为最后的选择。

缓解急迫性尿失禁症状的"膀胱训练"

"膀胱训练"的目的是训练大脑能够"坚持憋尿"的时间越来越长。这会使患者的症状从"尿急"变成痛苦的"憋尿"，往往会超过患者的忍耐程度。

膀胱或直肠脱垂的传统手术方式

这些"自体组织修补"的手术方式有 100 多年的历史，就是简单地切除阴道壁的膨出部分，再把切缘两边缝合在一起。受损组织吻合的依然是受损组织。这就解释了为什么膀胱膨出和直肠膨出修补术的治愈率通常都很低。此外，阴道是一个圆柱体，所以任何阴道壁组织的切除只会缩窄或缩短它，会潜在地导致性交问题。我们曾经见到过一例经过 3 次手术后阴道缩小至拇指大小的病例。这就是为什么大多数手术医生建议在手术中尽可能少地切除阴道组织。如果韧带是完好的，那么这些手术可以达到令人满意的效果。然而，脱垂的患者通常韧带也存在损伤，这就解释了此类手术成功率低的原因。

Traditional Surgery for Uterine Prolapse

The uterus can be conserved ("Manchester Repair") or removed (hysterectomy). Because we believe that the uterus plays a major part in maintaining organ support and because hysterectomy is a major operation with significant complications, we recommend not removing the uterus wherever possible. Furthermore, after removal of the uterus, the upper part of vagina often bulges down, like a glove turning inside out, because the ligaments which support it are weakened by the hysterectomy.

Vaginal Mesh Reinforcement Surgery for Prolapse

In the past 10 years, many surgeons have implanted large polypropylene mesh sheets below the vaginal wall. The meshes do not repair damaged ligaments. They work by blocking the bladder and bowel from protruding into the vagina. The problem with implanting a large sheet of foreign plastic material is that the body may react against it with varying degrees of intensity, ranging from nothing to swelling, redness, pain and scar tissue. The process is very similar to what happens with a splinter. Though mesh improves the surgical cure rate with prolapse surgery, it has, in some patients, caused pain with intercourse, smelly vaginal discharge, bladder and bowel perforations (fistulas) and other complications. This method has become sufficiently controversial to provoke warnings from the FDA, the American control agency. These mesh methods do not repair specific ligaments, so they cannot reliably cure symptoms.

Laparoscopic or Robotic Mesh Surgery

These operations are performed inside the abdominal peritoneal cavity. Robotic surgery is essentially the same as laparoscopic surgery, except that it is more expensive and takes longer to perform. Long 4 – 5 cm wide strips of mesh, equivalent in size to vaginal meshes, are attached to the upper part of the sacrum (tail

子宫脱垂的传统手术方式

子宫可以被保留（"曼彻斯特手术"），也可以被切除（子宫切除术）。我们之所以建议无论什么情况下都尽可能不要切除子宫，是因为我们相信子宫在维持器官支持方面起着重要的作用，而且子宫切除术是一个有并发症的大手术。此外，因为子宫切除后支撑阴道顶端的韧带被削弱，阴道顶端往往会向下膨出，就像手套被翻过来一样。

治疗脱垂的阴道网片加强手术

在过去的十多年里，许多外科医生在阴道壁下方置入了聚丙烯网片。该网片不能修复受损的韧带，它们通过阻止膀胱和肠道突向阴道而起作用。置入大块外来合成材料的问题是，人体可能会对其产生不同程度的排异反应，从没有任何反应到肿胀、发红、疼痛和瘢痕组织增生。这与被扎到木刺后的反应非常相似。网片可以提高脱垂手术的治愈率，但在一些患者中，网片会导致性交痛、阴道分泌物有异味、膀胱和肠穿孔（瘘管）等并发症。这种治疗方法引起了大量争议，为此，美国食品药品监督管理局（FDA）已经发出警告。这些置入网片的手术方法不能修复相应的韧带，因此不能可靠地缓解症状。

腹腔镜或机器人网片手术

这些手术是在腹腔内进行的。机器人手术本质上和腹腔镜手术一样，只是费用更高，手术时间更长。大小与阴道网片相当的 4～5 cm 宽的长条形网片，被分别附着于骶骨（尾骨）上部和

bone) and the upper part of the vagina. Usually the uterus has to be removed, potentially causing other problems, as outlined elsewhere in this book. The mesh creates an artificial back ligament. If correctly applied, the results for prolapse and symptoms can be quite good. However, like any foreign implanted material, severe tissue reaction can occur, in about 2% of cases. Such complications can sometimes be severe and may include bowel obstruction and dense adhesions. If the mesh is applied too tightly, it may cause problems with bladder and bowel emptying.

Stress Incontinence Surgery

Between 1960 and 2000, stress urinary incontinence was cured by operations which involved a large abdominal incisions. These operations cured stress incontinence reasonably well but were painful, patients could not pass urine after the operation and they required 10 – 14 day hospital stays.
In 1995, the midurethral sling (TVT) revolutionized stress incontinence surgery. A loop of tape inserted around the front ligament reduced stress incontinence surgery to a fairly painless one hospital day stay. Up to a 90% cure rate can be expected. The FDA has issued no warnings against TVT-type slings.

The Next Step—Use of "Minislings" for Prolapse and Incontinence

"Minisling" operations insert small strips of tape to reinforce damaged tissues. They are being increasingly used for the treatment of urinary stress incontinence. Adjustable ' minislings ' appear to be more effective than the standard variety which rely only on being pushed up to work. The TFS (Tissue Fixation System), an adjustable sling technique, was the first ' minisling '. It was performed in 2003 in patients from the Kvinno Centre. It became commercially available in 2009, having undergone rigorous testing for safety and efficacy over a period of 5 years before commercial release. It is the only ' minisling ' which can repair prolapses. It uses an identical philosophy to the TVT: small strips

阴道上部,这类手术通常需要切除子宫,如本书其他部分所述,这可能会引起其他问题。这个网片形成了一个人工的后部韧带。如果应用正确,脱垂和症状的治疗结果可以相当好。然而,与任何外来置入材料一样,约 2% 的病例会发生严重的组织反应。这种并发症有时很严重,可能包括肠梗阻和致密粘连。如果网片太紧,可能会导致膀胱和肠道排空异常的问题。

压力性尿失禁手术

1960 年至 2000 年间,压力性尿失禁通过腹式大切口手术治疗。这些手术治疗压力性尿失禁效果尚可,但患者也很痛苦,术后不能排尿,需要住院 10~14 天。

1995 年,尿道中段悬吊术(TVT)彻底改变了压力性尿失禁的手术方式。通过在前部韧带周围置入一环形吊带使得压力性尿失禁手术变得几乎没有痛苦,并且住院时间减少到一天。预期手术治愈率可达 90%。FDA 没有对 TVT 吊带发出警示。

下一阶段——应用"迷你吊带"治疗脱垂和尿失禁

"迷你吊带"手术通过放入小段吊带来强化受损组织。它们越来越多地被用于治疗压力性尿失禁。可调节性"迷你吊带"手术似乎比标准手术方式更有效,后者仅依赖于吊带的支持作用。组织固定系统(TFS)是一种可调节的吊带技术,是第一个"迷你吊带",2003 年首次应用于 Kvinno 中心的患者,在经过 5 年严格的安全性和有效性评估后于 2009 年上市,是唯一能修复脱垂的"迷你吊带"。它使用了与 TVT 手术相同的原理:用小段的条带支撑受损的韧带来治疗膀胱、直肠和子宫脱垂。TFS 的革

of tape support damaged ligaments to cure cystocele, rectocele and prolapse of the uterus. What is revolutionary about the TFS is that it also tightens loose ligaments, thereby restoring muscle strength.

It is this dual action which cures or improves many symptoms which were not previously considered as being curable, urgency, nocturia, frequency, pelvic pain, abnormal emptying, bowel incontinence and constipation. It also cures urinary stress incontinence equivalent to the TVT in the longer term.

Though minimally invasive and significantly safer than previous operations, 'minislings' are not complication free. The organs they seek to repair can be injured, usually during dissection and they are susceptible to all potential complications of implanted materials, including pain, excess tissue reaction and rejection in up to 3% of cases.

Pelvic Floor Exercises

We emphasize that the aim of the book and this section is to inform, not to advise treatment. Sensibly used, the exercises described are effective. However, as it is possible for spinal or other problems to cause harm, it is suggested that the exercises be performed under professional supervision.

Traditional Pelvic Floor Exercises were introduced by Dr Kegel in 1946. Kegel exercises do not actually cure stress incontinence. They train a bowel muscle, the puborectalis muscle to "squeeze upwards" to close the urethra immediately before a cough or sneeze. The patient must consciously squeeze upwards to prevent leakage. If this is done in time, the maneouvre is effective and it controls leakage. If not, the patient leaks.

Ideally, the woman should set some time aside, sit quietly, concentrate and lift up her pelvic muscles repeatedly. This is why there is such a large dropout rate with pelvic floor exercises- the woman just cannot find the time to fit them in! These Kegel exercises mainly strengthen the muscle which "cuts off" the urine, the puborectalis. They do not strengthen the backward acting muscles and ligaments which control other symptoms such as pain, urgency, nocturia (getting up at night) bowel and bladder emptying. These muscles can only be strengthened with

新之处在于它还能收紧松弛的韧带，从而恢复肌肉力量。正是这种双重作用治愈或改善了许多以前认为不可治愈的症状，如尿急、夜尿症、尿频、盆腔疼痛、排空异常、大便失禁和便秘。从长远来看，它治疗压力性尿失禁的疗效和 TVT 相当。

虽然"迷你吊带"手术比传统手术更加微创和安全，但它并不是没有并发症。在手术的过程中，它可能会损伤到目标脏器，同时也容易发生置入材料的所有可能的并发症，包括疼痛、过度组织反应和高达 3％的排异反应率。

盆底训练

我们强调，本书和这一节的目的是告知，而不是建议治疗。若应用合理，则所描述的训练是有效的。但是，由于可能损伤脊柱或造成其他问题，建议在专业人士监督下进行。

1946 年，凯格尔（Kegel）医生引入了传统的盆底训练。Kegel 的训练方法并不能真正治愈压力性尿失禁。该方法训练患者在即将咳嗽或打喷嚏前"向上收紧"肠道肌肉、耻骨直肠肌以关闭尿道。患者必须有意识地向上收紧以防止漏尿，如果能及时做到这一点，那么这个动作是有效的，并能控制漏尿；如果不及时，那患者依然会漏尿。

理想情况下，女性应该留出一些时间，安静地坐着，集中精力，反复地向上收紧骨盆肌肉。这就是为什么如此多的人进行盆底训练会半途而废——女性就是找不到时间来训练！Kegel 的训练方法主要是加强"中止"排尿的耻骨直肠肌。但 Kegel 的训练方法不能加强向后作用的肌肉和韧带，这些肌肉和韧带可以控制其他症状，如疼痛、尿急、夜尿症（晚上起床排尿）、肠道和膀胱排空。这些肌肉只能通过下面详细介绍的蹲式训练来加强。

squatting-based exercises as detailed below.

New Pelvic Floor Exercises based on the Integral System work differently. The "squatting culture" on which they are based strengthens the natural muscles and ligaments, so no conscious effort to close the urethra before a cough is required. Other symptoms such as pelvic pain, urgency and bladder emptying problems are also improved. Up to a 60% improvement is possible in 60% of symptoms in younger women using these methods. The way these muscles work is that they strengthen the pelvic muscles and the ligaments against which the muscles contract. We have found that these pelvic floor methods do not work so well with older women, because their ligaments are often too badly damaged to be strengthened in this way. Indeed, we have found that in a small percentage of cases (5%), stress incontinence symptoms may actually worsen with these methods. In such cases, a midurethral sling restores continence.

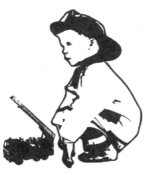

Fig 3 – 1. Zero time expended pelvic floor exercises—developing a "squatting culture"

"Squatting culture"—a simple time efficient method Rather than bending, the woman should train herself, as a daily routine, to squat down to pick up things. Examples are: using a dust pan, playing with a child, etc. An excellent adjunct is to use a rubber fitball instead of a chair at work. These are not so much exercises, as a better usage of muscles. They are very time efficient, as they become part of the daily routine. They can be reasonably effective in younger women but are not so helpful in older patients.

The Integral System exercises are based on squatting. The child squatting to pick up up a ball indicates that squatting is a fundamental human posture. Different cultures squat to eat, prepare meals, give birth, defaecate and urinate. Squatting has been scientifically proven to strengthen the natural muscles and ligaments, those needed to defecate, urinate and to control

基于"整体理论系统"的新型盆底训练有着不同的作用。该方法所基于的"蹲式文化"强化了肌肉和韧带，因此在咳嗽之前不需要有意识地闭合尿道。其他症状如盆腔疼痛、急迫感和膀胱排空问题也得到改善。在使用这些方法的年轻女性中，60％的症状可以获得高达60％程度的改善。这些肌肉的工作方式是能够加强骨盆肌肉和肌肉收缩所依赖的韧带。我们发现，这些盆底训练方法对老年妇女的效果不是太好，因为她们的韧带通常已经严重受损，无法用这种方法加强。事实上，我们发现，在一小部分病例（5％）中，这些方法反而可能加重压力性尿失禁症状。此时，应用尿道中段悬吊术可以恢复自控能力。

　　"蹲式文化"——相较弯腰而言的一种简单、省时的方法，女性应该在日常生活中养成下蹲捡东西的习惯，例如在使用簸箕、与孩子玩耍时，等等。一个很好的辅助手段是在工作时使用健身球代替椅子。与其说这些是锻炼，不如说是更好地利用肌肉。这些措施非常有效，因为它们会成为日常生活的一部分，对年轻女性相当有效，但对老年患者没有那么大的帮助（见图3-1）。

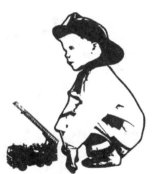

图3-1　不花时间的盆底训练——推行"蹲式文化"

　　"整体理论系统"的练习是以蹲姿为基础的。孩子蹲着捡球，说明下蹲是人的一种基本姿势。不同文化的人会蹲着吃饭、做饭、分娩、排便和排尿。科学证明，蹲姿可以增强自然肌肉和韧带，这些肌肉和韧带是排便、排尿和自控力所必需的。这些肌肉运动与"Kegel训练"的肌肉运动完全不同，它们不是自然的，需要学习。我们不提倡重复下蹲练习。准确地说，我们建议弯

continence. These muscle movements are quite different to the "Kegel" muscles which are not natural and need to be taught. We are not advocating repetitive squatting exercises. Rather we recommend bending the knees to pick something up instead of bending down with knees straight. This is a zero time exercise that should become part of daily life.

If it is possible to perform daily tasks in the squatting position (as some tribal women do), so much the better.

In the developing foetus, the abdominal muscles and pelvic muscles originate from the same place. Therefore any exercise which strengthens the abdominal muscles also strengthens the pelvic muscles. Situps with bent knees automaticaly strengthen the pelvic muscles and ligaments. These take literally $2 - 3$ seconds for each situp. Often only 2 or 3 situps are possible when starting. However, progress is rapid and the effect on pelvic floor symptoms and chronic back pain is often remarkable. It is wise to check with your doctor before starting any such exercises.

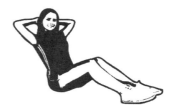

Fig $3 - 2$ (Almost) zero time expended pelvic floor exercises—situps prior to getting out of bed

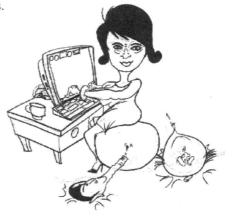

Fig $3 - 3$ More zero time expended pelvic floor exercises. "···and it also fixed my back

曲膝盖来捡东西,而不是膝盖绷直弯腰下来。这是一个不花费时间的运动,应该成为日常生活的一部分(见图3-2)。

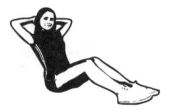

图3-2 (几乎)不花时间的盆底训练——起床前仰卧起坐

如果能像一些部落妇女那样,以蹲姿完成日常工作,那就更好了。

在胎儿发育中,腹肌和盆底肌肉的起源是相同的。因此,任何增强腹部肌肉的运动也会增强骨盆肌肉。膝关节自动弯曲的仰卧起坐可以加强骨盆肌肉和韧带。每次仰卧起坐真的只需要2~3秒。刚开始的时候患者通常只能做2个或3个仰卧起坐。然而,随着训练的加强,她们进步迅速,盆底症状和慢性背痛的改善往往是显著的。在开始任何这样的锻炼之前,患者最好先咨询一下自己的医生(见图3-3)。

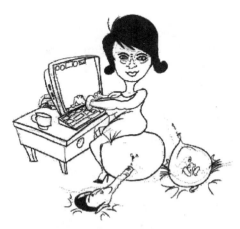

图3-3 更多不花时间的盆底训练。"……而且它还治好了我的背痛

The pelvic floor is composed of two types of muscle, fast-twitch and slow-twitch. Slow-twitch muscles are by far the most common. Whereas the fast-twitch muscles are important for sudden stresses such as sneezing, sitting on a rubber fitball instead of a chair at work or at home automatically strengthens the slow-twitch muscles which prevent urine and bowel leaking on a continual basis. The abdominal, back and pelvic floor muscles are also strengthened.

Which patients are most suitable for pelvic floor exercises?

As a generalization, the younger the patient, the less the damage inflicted on the muscles and ligaments by childbirth and age, the better the result. That said, we have seen good results in some older patients. Our view is that it is worthwhile for any motivated patient to try these methods, irrespective of her age.

What if I cannot squat?

Situps are still possible and perhaps the rubber fitball, but only if the woman has retained a good sense of balance.

During pregnancy

Kegel exercises, (squeezing upwards) are standard for pregnancy and are recommended. Other than sitting on a fitball which imposes no strain, we advise strongly against the squatting-based exercises discussed above during pregnancy, because the Relaxin hormone weakens the ligaments considerably, so they may not be able to sustain the forces imposed upon them by squatting-type exercises. It is best to wait at least 6 weeks after giving birth before a "squatting-based" regime is undertaken.

Further information on surgical and non-surgical treatments is

盆底由快肌纤维和慢肌纤维两种肌肉组成。到目前为止,慢肌纤维的肌肉最常见。而快肌纤维的肌肉对于突发的压力如打喷嚏很重要,在工作或家里坐在健身球而不是椅子上,会自动加强慢肌纤维的肌肉,从而逐渐防止尿漏和粪漏。腹部、背部和盆底的肌肉也能得到加强。

哪些患者最适合盆底训练?

概括来说,患者越年轻,分娩和年龄对肌肉和韧带造成的损伤越小,盆底训练的效果也越好。尽管如此,我们在一些老年患者身上也还是看到了良好的效果。我们的观点是,无论年龄大小,任何有意向的患者都值得尝试这些训练方法。

如果我不能下蹲怎么办?

我们仍然可以进行仰卧起坐,也可以尝试健身球,但前提是妇女须拥有良好的平衡感。

怀孕期间

凯格尔(Kegel)训练(向上收紧)是怀孕期间推荐进行的标准训练。除了坐在一个不会产生压力的健身球上,我们强烈建议不要在怀孕期间进行上述蹲式运动,因为松弛素大大地削弱了韧带,它们可能无法承受蹲式运动所施加的压力。最好在分娩至少 6 周后再采取"蹲式"训练体系。

更多有关手术治疗和保守治疗的信息,请访问 www.integrantheory.org 或医学教科书《女性骨盆底——基于整体理论功能、功能障碍及管理》(第三版)的第四章和第五章,该书由

available at www. integraltheory. org or in Chapters 4 and 5 of the medical textbook. " The Female Pelvic Floor, Function, Dysfunction and Management According to the Integral System", PEP Petros, 3rd Edition, Springer Heidelberg 2010.

Stories from the clinic

The three chapters which follow describe a range of case histories from patients who were treated with repair of ligaments in the front, middle and back parts of the vagina, mainly with the TFS system. These chapters are all based on the experience of the authors. If any of the cases described in the chapters which follow bear a similarity to your problem, we suggest you discuss the particular case history with your doctor.

PEP Petros 著,2010 年经施普林格出版社(海德堡)出版。

临床病例

接下来的三章讲述了一系列阴道前部、中部、后部韧带修补的病例,大部分都应用了 TFS 系统。这些章节都是基于作者们的经验。如果以下章节中描述的任何病例与您的症状相似,我们建议您与医生讨论个人病史。

(上海交通大学医学院附属第六人民医院妇产科,李毓 译,薛卓维 校)

CHAPTER 4   Is This Your Problem?
—Front ligament damage

In this section, we give a series of testimonies from patients who came to our clinic with particular problems caused by front ligament looseness.

Stress incontinence (leaking during coughing, sneezing, exercise) is the main symptom for front ligament looseness.

Other front ligament symptoms include urgency when associated with stress incontinence and faecal incontinence when associated with stress incontinence and urine loss during intercourse.

Stress Incontinence from Front Ligament Looseness

Mrs CYL, was 55 years old and she had had 3 normal deliveries. She had chronic bronchitis, and she gave this story.
"I was at a cocktail party with my husband. It was a special occasion and I was wearing my new long gown. I started coughing. It was terribly embarrassing. The urine just ran down my leg and it wouldn't stop. I left a trail of urine on the carpet. I wanted the earth to open and swallow me. Previously, I hadn't wanted to go to the doctor, because my sister had a big operation for the same thing. She had all sorts of problems after the operation. She couldn't pass urine for a month and she had to learn to self-catheterize. Even now she has to lean forward to pass urine and wait, and go again. She still has incontinence. I had managed to cope in the past by going very frequently to the toilet

第四章　您有这样的问题吗？
——前部韧带损伤

在本章中，我们列举了一系列在我们诊所就诊的前部韧带松弛患者的自述。

压力性尿失禁（表现为咳嗽、打喷嚏、运动时漏尿）**是前部韧带松弛的主要症状。**

其他前部韧带症状包括与压力性尿失禁相关的尿急，与压力性尿失禁相关的粪失禁和性交中的漏尿。

前部韧带松弛引起的压力性尿失禁

CYL 太太，55 岁，正常分娩 3 次。患有慢性支气管炎，她讲述了以下这个故事：

"有一次，我和丈夫一起去参加一个鸡尾酒会，那是一个特殊的场合，我穿着新的长裙。当我开始咳嗽时，无比尴尬的事情发生了，尿液顺着两腿不停地流下来，在地毯上留下了一小撮尿痕。我真希望找个地洞钻进去。以前，我不想去看医生，因为我姐姐由于同样的症状接受了一次大手术，但术后出现了各种各样的问题：她一个月无法正常排尿，不得不学会自我导尿。即使是现在，在排尿时也必须身体前倾，停顿一会，然后再反复进行此动作。而且她依然有尿失禁。过去，我经常去洗手间提前排空膀胱以应付这种情况。在鸡尾酒会之后，丈夫建议我至少

to empty my bladder. After the cocktail party episode, my husband suggested I at least go and talk to my doctor. I told the doctor about my sister. He said there was a new technique which didn't cause much pain or problems with passing water, and he said he would refer me to a clinic which specialized in this method".

Mrs CYL had our standard assessment, which confirmed that the damage was in the front ligament. We were amazed to find that she was leaking almost one third of her normal urine output into large incontinence pads. The ultrasound showed that her bladder and urethra became one large funnel when she coughed and the urine just ran out.

We explained to her that stress incontinence denotes looseness in the front ligament. The operation was simple. A small length of polypropylene tape was inserted through a very small incision in the vagina and placed in the exact position of the front ligament. The patient went home the next day entirely dry. Prior to surgery all potential problems likely to be encountered were discussed in detail. We explained that the main problem with these operations is rejection of the tape by the body in $2-5\%$ of cases, much in the manner of a splinter. We explained that generally this is a minor complication, which can be dealt without admission to hospital, simply by trimming the tape.

Stress and Urge Incontinence from Front Ligament Looseness

When urge occurs along with stress incontinence, it is called ssion to hospital,". Urgency may occur with looseness in any part of the vagina, front, middle or back. In the case which follows, the cause of the urgency and stress incontinence was loosenessin the front ligament.

Mrs JC was a typically busy 38 year old lady, just coping with 2 young children, a husband, a home, and a part-time job. She had

去看一次医生。我把姐姐的情况告诉了医生。他说,有一种新技术不会给排尿造成太大的痛苦或问题,随后把我转至专门研究这种方法的诊所。

CYL太太接受了标准评估,证实了损伤位于前部韧带。令我们吃惊的是,她几乎将1/3的正常尿量漏到尿垫中。超声检查显示,她在咳嗽时,膀胱和尿道连接部会形成漏斗样改变,从而发生漏尿。

我们向她解释,压力性尿失禁是由于前部韧带松弛所致。手术很简单。将一小段聚丙烯吊带通过阴道上的一个很小的切口置入,并放置在前部韧带的相应位置。第二天患者就能完全控制小便,康复出院了。在手术之前,我们详细讨论了所有可能遇到的潜在风险。这一手术的主要风险是会有2%～5%的患者发生吊带排异,类似木刺扎到后的反应。这是一个较轻的并发症,只需修剪外露的吊带即可解决,而无须住院。

前部韧带松弛引起的压力性和急迫性尿失禁

当急迫性尿失禁与压力性尿失禁同时发生时,被称为"混合性尿失禁"。阴道前部、中部或后部的任何部位发生松弛,均会出现尿急症状。下面所描述的病例中,急迫性和压力性尿失禁的原因是前部韧带松弛。

JC太太,38岁,是一个忙碌的女士,需要照顾两个小孩、丈夫和家庭,她还有一份兼职工作。她患有压力性尿失禁,并且每天会在到达厕所前因尿急而漏尿2～3次。她说:

"我去看了另一位医生,他说他不会为我做压力性尿失禁手术,因为我的尿动力学检测*显示是"不稳定性膀胱",手术后会加重尿急症状。他们给我使用药物治疗,但由于不良反应而

stress incontinence and she also wet herself with urgency 2 – 3 times a day before she arrived at the toilet. She said,

"I went to another doctor who said he would not operate for my tress incontinence because the urodynamic test * *showed I had an dunstable bladder".* *I was told that my urgency would get worse with the surgery. They put me on drug treatment, which I had to stop because of the side effects. My mouth became so dry. I became constipated and I couldn't empty my bladder properly."*

Her previous medical advice had made her very cautious about undergoing surgery. We were able to convince Mrs JC that her front ligament was causing both her stress and urge, by gently pressing a finger upwards on one side just behind the pubic bone. This controlled her urine loss on coughing and greatly diminished her urge symptoms. She was cured of both stress and urge with a small segment of tape placed around the middle of her urethra to strengthen the front ligament.

* A Urodynamics test measures the pressures in the bladder.

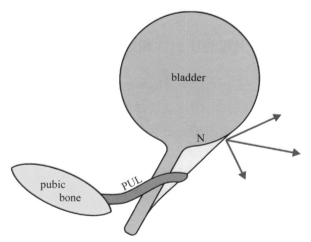

Fig 4 – 1   How a loose front ligament caused stress and urge incontinence in Mrs JC

不得不停药,不良反应包括口干、便秘和排尿不净感。"

以往的医疗经历使她对再次手术非常谨慎。通过用手指轻轻地在耻骨后方的一侧阴道壁向上按压,控制了她在咳嗽时的漏尿和尿急症状后,我们成功地说服了 JC 太太,使她认识到前部韧带松弛是压力性和急迫性尿失禁共同的原因。她接受了在尿道中段放置一小段吊带以加强前部韧带的手术,同时治愈了压力性和急迫性尿失禁。

*尿动力学检查测量膀胱压力。

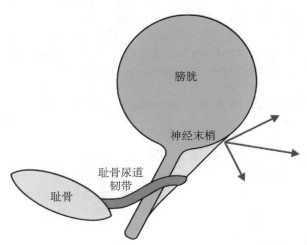

图 4 - 1　前部韧带松弛如何导致 JC 太太的压力性尿失禁和急迫性尿失禁

A loose front ligament "PUL", cannot support the urethral tube, so the tube is pulled open during a cough by the pelvic muscles (arrows), thereby causing urine leakage, known as stress incontinence. Neither can a loose "PUL" support the nerve endings "N" (stretch receptors), so they send off signals to the brain, which interprets them as urge symptoms. A tape placed at "PUL", the front ligament, provides support for the urethral tube and "N", to cure both the stress and urge incontinence.

Women such as Mrs JC can expect up to a 90% cure rate for their stress incontinence and a 50 – 60% cure rate for their urgency symptoms. Those women who continue to have urge symptoms after repair of the front ligaments, most likely have looseness in some other ligament. For example, if they also have pelvic pain, get up at night a few times to pass urine or cannot empty properly, it is likely that their back ligaments are also loose (see chapter 6).

Comment on urgency associated with stress urinary incontinence

We have seen many patients such as Mrs JC, who, because of associated urgency, have been refused treatment even for their stress incontinence. This is a hangover from past attitudes. Fortunately, an increasing number of doctors are now accepting that both stress and urge can be cured with a tape which reinforces the front ligament.

Urine Loss with Sexual Intercourse

Mrs DB, a 28 year old lady came to us with this story.
"*We were childhood sweethearts. We married early and worked hard to buy our little house. Three months ago, a beautiful little boy came along to fill our lives. We were so happy. My husband and I always had a good sex life and he just couldn't wait to start again. Six weeks after the baby we had sex for the first time. Soon*

松弛的前部韧带"耻骨尿道韧带（PUL）"无法支撑尿道，因此咳嗽时，盆腔的肌力（图4-1箭头所示）将其拉开，导致漏尿，这被称为压力性尿失禁。同样，松弛的"耻骨尿道韧带"也不能支持神经末梢"N"（牵张感受器），它们向大脑发送排尿信号，导致尿急症状。在前部韧带"耻骨尿道韧带（PUL）"处放置一条吊带，可以支撑尿道和神经末梢"N"，同时治疗压力性和急迫性尿失禁。

像JC太太这样的患者，预期压力性尿失禁的治愈率高达90％，而尿急症状的治愈率为50％～60％。那些在阴道前部韧带修复后仍有尿急症状的女性，很可能还存在其他韧带的松弛。例如，如果合并盆腔疼痛、多次夜尿或排尿不净感，其后部韧带也可能存在松弛（请参阅第六章）。

对压力性尿失禁伴有尿急症状的点评

我们见过很多像JC太太这样的患者，由于伴有尿急症状，医生拒绝治疗压力性尿失禁。这主要是基于医生对以往临床病例的认识。幸运的是，现在越来越多的医生开始认可压力性尿失禁和急迫性尿失禁都可以通过（尿道中段）吊带来加强前部韧带而获得治愈。

性生活中的漏尿症状

DB太太，28岁，给我们带来了下面这个故事：

"我和丈夫青梅竹马，很早就结婚了，并努力工作购买了一套小房子。3个月前，一个漂亮的小男孩出现在我们的生活中，我们非常高兴。之前，我和丈夫的性生活一直很和谐，他迫不及待地想要重新开始。孩子出生6周后，我们第一次做爱。我们

after we started, I felt this warm fluid pouring over my thighs and into the bed. My husband stopped and said "What's this?". It was urine. It happened again the next night and every night we tried. We went back to our gynaecologist who said he didn't know what the problem was, but it might be helped with pelvic floor exercises. I went to a physio who taught me how to squeeze up my pelvic floor muscles. I tried it for a month. It sort of worked sometimes, but I was so anxious now, that I just couldn't bring myself to have sex any more. "

We had seen several such women, all of whom had been cured by inserting a sling to repair the front ligament. One concern with Mrs DB was that she wanted to have another baby. We were able to assure her that this would not be a problem and she would not need a Caesarian Section. Six weeks after the operation, Mrs DB and her husband had their first intercourse. She rang to tell us the next day that everything was now fine and that she was cured.

Comment

Leaking urine during intercourse may have tragic consequences, even marriage breakup. One method which often works is to squeeze upwards as the penis thrusts in (Kegel exercise). This action pulls up the vagina and prevents the penis from opening out the bladder tube (urethra). It also enhances pleasure for both parties. If this does not work, a sling, as is used for stress incontinence, can cure the problem. If there is also pain during intercourse, the consequences for the marriage may be even worse, as often nothing is found on investigation and the husband may feel it is the woman's way of avoiding intercourse. Therefore, many women choose to suffer the pain silently, another Conspiracy of Silence. This condition may be caused by loose ligaments and can occur even in young women who have not had children.

开始后不久,我就感觉有股温热的液体从大腿流到床上。我丈夫停下来问:"这是什么?"是尿!第二天晚上又发生了同样的事,每次都是这样。我的妇科医生说他不知道问题出在什么地方,但是盆底肌肉锻炼可能会有所帮助。一位理疗师教我如何收缩盆底肌肉,我试了 1 个月。有时候有点效果,但是我现在很焦虑,根本不想再做爱了。"

我们见过几名这样的女性,她们都通过置入吊带修复前部韧带而获得治愈。DB 太太的顾虑是她还想要一个孩子。我们向她保证,这不是个问题,也不需要因此而行剖宫产。术后 6 周,DB 太太和她的丈夫进行了手术后的第一次性生活。第二天她告诉我们,现在一切都很好,她已经痊愈了。

点 评

性生活时漏尿可能会导致悲剧性后果,甚至导致婚姻破裂。通常有效的方法是在阴茎插入时盆底肌肉向上收缩（Kegel 训练）。该动作可收紧阴道并防止阴茎打开尿道,还可增加双方的性愉悦。如果这样不起作用,则可采用治疗压力性尿失禁的吊带进行治疗。如果性交时还感到疼痛,婚姻的后果可能会更糟,因为往往难以找到任何病因,丈夫会觉得这是女方回避性生活的手段。因此,许多女性选择默默地忍受痛苦,这是另一种"缄默的密约"。事实上,这种情况可能是韧带松弛引起的,甚至在未生育孩子的年轻女性中也可能发生。

Urge Incontinence Dating from Childhood Caused by a Loose Front Ligament

In some cases, weak front ligaments may cause childhood urgency. Miss 'A', a 21 year old single woman, came to the clinic with her mother. She was shy, teary and withdrawn. She gave this story.

"Since childhood, I have not been able to control my bladder. I always wear pads and I always smell of urine. Every time I go out on a date, I am terrified that my companion will smell the urine. I am sure I have lost several boy friends in this way. The whole thing is extremely distressing and humiliating. I'd rather stay home than go out and be embarrassed. "

Our diagnostic system indicated that a weak front ligament was the main cause of her problems. The weak ligament was obvious on ultrasound. When we pressed gently upwards on the vagina immediately behind the bone, all the feelings of urgency disappeared, confirming that a weak front ligament was causing her urge symptoms. A polypropylene tape was inserted in the position of the front ligament. Immediately after surgery Miss 'A' reported 100% dryness. She remained cured at her last review 4 years later, where a happy confident young woman arrived, accompanied by a doting fiance.

Comment as to why women who have not been pregnant can develop incontinence

In chapters 1 & 2 we discussed how ligaments stretched loose by childbirth caused incontinence and prolapse. Some women are born with loose ligaments and so they may suffer problems from childhood.

因前部韧带松弛而导致的儿童急迫性失禁

在某些情况下,前部韧带薄弱可能会导致儿童尿急症状。
21 岁的单身女性 A 小姐和她母亲一起来到诊所。她很害羞,沉
默寡言,默默流泪。她告诉我们这个故事:

"自小时候起,我就无法控制自己的膀胱。我总是佩戴
尿垫,身上总有尿味。每次出去约会,我都害怕同伴会闻到
身上的尿味。我确信已经有几个男朋友因此离开我。整个
事情令人极其沮丧和羞愧。我宁愿待在家里,也不愿出门受
窘。"

我们的诊断系统表明,前部韧带薄弱是她出现问题的主要
原因。超声检查也显示其韧带薄弱。当我们轻轻向上按压耻骨
后面的阴道时,所有的急迫感都消失了,这证明前部韧带薄弱导
致了她的尿急症状。我们在手术中将一根聚丙烯吊带置入其
前部韧带的位置,手术后 A 小姐立即反馈说达到了 100% 的
控尿。在 4 年后的最后一次随访中,她仍然没有漏尿。这时
的她是一位快乐而自信的年轻女子,带着宠爱她的未婚夫一
起来到诊室。

关于为什么没有生育的女性会出现尿失禁的点评

在第一章和第二章中,我们讨论了韧带因分娩而松弛导致
尿失禁和脱垂的情况。但一些女性天生就有韧带松弛,她们可
能从童年开始就经历着痛苦。

Bedwetting from Childhood Caused by a Lax Front Ligament

Miss M, a 25 year old woman, came to us because a GP she consulted informed her that our clinic was using a new method which had helped some of her patients who had difficult problems. She stated:

"I wet my bed as a child. They took me to the doctor who said it was "behavioural". Every time I wet my bed, I was belted by my parents who said I was doing it deliberately. When I reached puberty, the bed wetting ceased but I still wet with coughing and exercise and I still couldn't control my bladder when I had the urge to go. When I was 19 years old, I had a bladder elevation operation. I had this great big scar right across my tummy. I couldn't pass urine for 2 weeks. I had so much pain even when I left the hospital two weeks later. The operation didn't work. I still wet when I coughed and I still wet during the day. I was always in and out of toilets".

There was a grimness about Miss M, the type of grim determination required to negotiate the harshness of her life and her condition. She was overweight, unsmiling but not aggressive or demanding. Ultrasound demonstrated that the front ligament was loose. Like Miss A, her bladder symptoms were cured with a sling which reinforced her front ligaments. Unlike Miss A, there was no dramatic change in her mood. The damage to her psyche was too deep-seated for that. She politely declined an offer for counselling, saying it was up to herself to get on with her life and she would be starting a fitness programme at her local gym as soon as the 3 month recovery period had been completed.

Comment Children who leak urine or wet their bed often become psychologically disturbed and may develop behavioural problems. It is unfortunate that some "researchers" get it back to front and say that it is the "behavioural problems" which are the cause of the bedwetting. These children should be loved and supported and told that the problem will settle once they reach puberty.

前部韧带松弛导致儿童遗尿

M小姐,25岁。之所以来找我们,是因为她的家庭医生告诉她,我们的诊所正在应用一种新的疗法,该方法已经帮助了一些遇到同样问题的患者。她说:

"我小时候就经常尿床。父母带我去看医生,医生说那是"儿童行为"。每次我尿床的时候,就会被父母体罚,他们觉得我是故意的。当我进入青春期后,就不尿床了,但是咳嗽和运动后仍会漏尿。在感到尿意需要上厕所时,我还会漏尿。19岁的时候,我做了膀胱颈抬高手术,肚子上留下了一个巨大的瘢痕。术后两周都无法排尿,即使两周后出院时,我仍感到非常疼痛。手术并没有明显效果,咳嗽时和白天还是会漏尿。我总是无法远离厕所。"

M小姐,表情严肃,流露出她直面窘迫的生活状况和病情所必备的坚毅。她体重超标,面无笑容,但不咄咄逼人也不苛刻。超声检查显示其前部韧带松弛。像A小姐一样,M小姐的膀胱症状通过置入吊带加强前部韧带而得到了治愈。不过与A小姐不同的是,她的情绪没有明显变化,可能是因为心灵受到了过往经历的深深伤害。她礼貌地拒绝了我们的建议,要主导自己的生活。她会在3个月的术后恢复期结束后,立即在她当地的健身房开始健身计划。

点评:漏尿或遗尿的孩子经常会内心不安,并可能因此出现行为问题。不幸的是,一些"研究者"弄反了顺序,认为"行为问题"是遗尿的原因。事实上,这些孩子应该受到关爱和心理支持,应该告诉他们进入青春期后问题就会得到解决。

Bedwetting from Childhood and Faecal incontinence Caused by a Lax Front Ligament

In contrast, Miss G, 18 years old, had an understanding mother. Miss G was reluctantly brought to the clinic by her mother who had heard about the clinic from a neighbour. She was sullen, resentful and aggressive to the staff. She had wet her bed since childhood and also had faecal incontinence. On examination, her urine loss was controlled by gentle pressure applied upwards in the vagina, just behind the pubic bone. She agreed to an ultrasound test. This indicated that she had a very loose front ligament. Fortunately, she responded to the explanations offered: her front ligaments were loose, the tape would repair them, the operation was minimal and virtually risk free and she had a real chance of being cured. At the 6 week post-operative visit, we saw a remarkable transformation. A charming smiling young woman bounced into the room and announced she was cured.

We have seen many patients like Ms G and Ms M with a particular condition which runs in families, even in male children: nocturnal enuresis (wetting the bed at night), daytime symptoms of urgency and often stress incontinence. There may be a mother, an aunt or uncle who had this problem as a child. The symptoms usually disappear or improve greatly after puberty, probably because the gush of hormones at puberty strengthens the front ligament.

Comment on bedwetting causation

Bedwetting is a complex subject with many potential causes. We emphasize that we are not proposing that all bedwetting is caused by loose front ligaments. Our experience concerns only those women with demonstrable looseness in the front ligaments who were diagnosed as adults. Whatever the cause, most bedwetting problems resolve at puberty. However, we have seen many young women continue with daytime bladder problems, even after their bedwetting had resolved at puberty.

前部韧带松弛导致的童年遗尿和粪失禁

相比之下，18 岁的 G 小姐有一位善解人意的母亲。G 小姐很不情愿地被母亲带到诊所（她母亲听邻居介绍过我们诊所）。她对我们的工作人员阴沉着脸，愤愤不平，咄咄逼人。她从小就尿床，还有大便失禁。检查发现，只要在耻骨后方的阴道向上轻轻施压，就可以控制漏尿。她同意做超声检查，结果表明其前部韧带非常松弛。我们向她解释：她的前部韧带松弛，可以用吊带将其修复，手术创伤很小，几乎没有风险，而且她很有可能被治愈。幸运的是，她选择接受手术治疗。在术后 6 周的随访中，我们看到了惊人的转变：一个迷人的年轻女子微笑着蹦进房间，宣布她已康复。

我们已经看过很多像 G 小姐和 M 小姐这样有着特殊病情的患者，遗尿（夜间尿床）常在很多家庭成员甚至是男孩中发生，他们白天经常出现急迫性和压力性尿失禁等特殊情况。家庭中的母亲、阿姨或叔叔都有可能在小时候存在这个问题。这些症状通常在青春期后消失或明显改善，可能是因为青春期喷涌的激素强化了其前部韧带所致。

关于遗尿病因的点评

遗尿是一个复杂的问题，有很多潜在病因。我们强调，并不是所有遗尿都是由前部韧带松弛所引起。我们的经验仅涉及那些已被证实为前部韧带明显松弛的成年妇女。无论原因是什么，大多数遗尿问题都会在青春期好转。但是，我们也观察到许多年轻妇女，她们即使青春期后不再遗尿，但白天仍会出现膀胱问题。

We have found that a very high rate of cure can be achieved by repairing the front ligament with a midurethral sling operation.

Urinary and Faecal Incontinence Caused by a Lax Front Ligament

Cure of faecal incontinence after reconstruction of the front ligament was an accidental discovery. In the early days of the clinic, we were unaware of this association. One day a 65 year old lady, Mrs KH, who had undergone an operation for cure of her stress incontinence came in smiling. We asked, "Is your bladder cured?" She shook her head slowly and said "no doctor, sorry to disappoint you. I'm still leaking a little urine but you have fixed my bowel". (Another example of the passive "Conspiracy of Silence"-she did not even tell her doctor she had faecal incontinence!) We said, said, tor she had fanything to the bowel." Mrs KH replied, "well, whatever you have done, you've fixed it". This was a surprising but welcome outcome. It was not unique. Subsequently, many other patients volunteered that both their bladder and bowel incontinence had been cured by the same procedure. The relationship of faecal incontinence to damaged ligaments was not finally established scientifically until September 2008, when a series of scientific articles was published. All these papers can be viewed free online at www. pelviperineology. org, September 2008.

Stress Faecal Incontinence Caused by a Lax Front Ligament

Mrs T, 45 years old, came to see us because she lost urine and solid faeces on coughing. Again, symptom grouping with stress urinary incontinence gave us the clue that her symptoms originated from front ligament damage. She had been a keen golfer but had to cease this and all other social activities. Her assessment

我们发现,通过尿道中段吊带手术修复前部韧带可以达到很高的治愈率。

前部韧带松弛导致的尿失禁和粪失禁

重建前部韧带后可以治疗粪失禁是一个意外的发现。在诊所成立之初,我们还没有意识到这一关联。有一天,65 岁的KH 太太,一位压力性尿失禁术后患者,面带微笑地前来复诊。我们问:"您的膀胱问题好了吗?"她慢慢地摇了摇头,说:"没有,医生,很抱歉让您失望了。我仍在漏尿,但我不漏大便了"(另一个被动"缄默的密约"的例证,她甚至没有告诉医生她患有粪失禁!)。我们说:"但是我们没有对直肠做任何处理。"KH 太太回答说:"好吧,不管您做了什么,这个问题解决了"。这是令人惊讶但也令人振奋的结果。她并不是唯一的病例。随后,许多其他患者自愿坦陈,相同的手术同时治愈了尿失禁和粪失禁。直到 2008 年 9 月我们的一系列科学论文发表后,粪失禁与韧带损伤的关系才算最终得到确立。所有这些论文都可在网站(www. pelviperineology. org)2008 年 9 月的那一期免费查看。

前部韧带松弛导致的压力性粪失禁

T 太太,45 岁。她来找我们,是因为咳嗽时漏尿合并漏固体粪便。同样,压力性尿失禁的症候群为我们提供了线索,她的症状可能源自前部韧带损伤。她曾经是一名热衷高尔夫球运动的人,但现在她必须停止这项活动以及所有其他社交活动。检查表明她的前部韧带已经受损,我们用聚丙烯吊带解决了该问题。当她来术后随访时,我们几乎认不出她:那个佝偻、头发凌

indicated she had damaged front ligaments which we addressed with a polypropylene sling. We hardly recognized her when she came for her post-operative visit. Instead of a stooped dishevelled woman, we saw a vital well-dressed woman holding a large bunch of flowers and she had already played her first game of golf.

Comment on the characteristics of faecal incontinence

Typical symptoms, in order of severity, are uncontrolled wind loss, liquid soiling and solid faecal soiling. There are two main categories: an anal sphincter torn at childbirth, which needs to be repaired and another where no obvious cause can be found. When no obvious cause can be found, it is called "idiopathic incontinence" and it is this type of incontinence which may be caused by damage to the front or back ligaments.

Comment on causation of faecal incontinence

The bowel works in a similar way to the bladder. This explains why bladder and bowel symptoms often occur simultaneously. If a ligament is loose, the muscles which close the bowel cannot work properly and the patient may leak wind, fluid or solid faeces.

乱的女人不见了,出现在我们面前的是一个衣着考究的女人。她捧着一大束鲜花前来致谢,告诉我们在术后她已经打了第一场高尔夫球。

对粪失禁特征的点评

按照严重程度,粪失禁的典型症状是不受控制的肛门排气、排稀便和成形粪便。主要分为两类:一类为分娩时肛门括约肌裂伤所致,需要手术修复;另一类找不到明确的原因,被称为"特发性粪失禁",这种类型的粪失禁可能是由前部韧带或后部韧带的损伤引起的。

对粪失禁病因的点评

肠道的工作原理与膀胱相似。这就解释了为什么膀胱和肠道症状经常同时发生。如果韧带松弛,则闭合肠管的肌肉将无法正常工作,稀便或固体粪便就会漏出。

(上海交通大学医学院附属仁济医院泌尿科,方伟林 译,吕坚伟 校)

CHAPTER 5   Is This Your Problem?
—Middle ligaments damage

Middle Ligament Damage

The main symptom is a lump coming down, known as bladder prolapse or cystocele. Often there is difficulty in emptying the bladder and sometimes there is urgency.

Recurrent or Chronic Cystitis—Its Relationship to Abnormal Emptying, Cystocele and Prolapse of the Uterus

Cystitis means infection in the bladder. There are many causes of cystitis. Our specific interest is in patients who have recurrent cystitis because they cannot empty their bladder adequately due to damaged ligaments in the middle or back parts of the vagina. In our experience, cystocele and prolapse of the uterus are major correctable causes of abnormal emptying and chronic bladder infections. Bladder infection is diagnosed by taking a clean midstream specimen of urine and culturing It for bacteria. Women are much more vulnerable than men, because the urethra is short, allowing easy entry of bacteria. In the younger woman, the urethra closes off efficiently, blocking entry of bacteria. The lining of their urethra is spongy, with many blood vessels and cells called macrophages, which "mop up" any stray bacteria. After the menopause, the lack of hormones causes the cells and blood vessels to shrink (atrophy). The collagen also loosens with age. All these changes facilitate the entry of bacteria.
If the patient cannot adequately empty her bladder, the urine which remains in the bladder encourages the bacteria to multiply, unhindered by the body's defence mechanisms.

第五章　您有这样的问题吗？
——中部韧带损伤

中部韧带损伤

主要症状是块物脱出，称为膀胱脱垂或膀胱膨出。通常表现为膀胱排空困难，有时会有尿急症状。

复发性或慢性膀胱炎——与膀胱排空异常、膀胱膨出及子宫脱垂的关系

膀胱炎是指膀胱的感染，可能由多种病因引起。需要我们重点关注的是，一些复发性膀胱炎是由于阴道中部或后部的韧带受损而无法充分排空膀胱所致。根据我们的经验，膀胱膨出和子宫脱垂是导致膀胱排空异常和慢性膀胱炎主要且可纠正的病因。膀胱感染可通过洁净的中段尿细菌培养来诊断。女性的尿道较短，细菌容易入侵，因而比男性更易罹患膀胱炎。年轻女子的尿道口能有效关闭，从而阻止细菌侵入。其尿道周围结缔组织呈海绵状，有丰富的血管和巨噬细胞，巨噬细胞可以"吞噬"散在的细菌。绝经后，由于激素缺乏引起细胞和血管的皱缩（萎缩），胶原蛋白也随年龄增长而松弛，所有这些变化均有助于细菌的入侵。

如果患者不能充分排空膀胱，膀胱中残留的尿液会促使细菌繁殖，对抗身体防御机制（见图 5-1）。

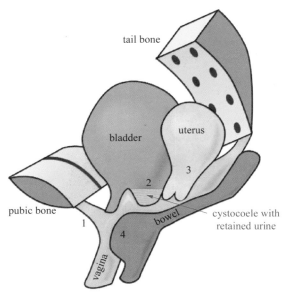

tail bone

uterus

bladder

3

2

pubic bone

bowel

cystocoele with
retained urine

1

4

vagina

Fig 5 – 1 **Cystocele with retained urine. The cystocele "2",**
droops downwards in a sac, preventing it from
emptying. The urine pool gets infected over time,
leading to chronic cystitis.

The first line of defence in the post-menopausal woman is to prescribe
a vaginally applied oestrogen tablet or cream, daily for 2 weeks, then
3 times weekly. Oestrogen restores the sponginess of the cells of the
vagina and urethra. Oestrogen given in this way acts mainly locally
and is not considered to cause any problems with breast cancer. We
recommend adequate fluids to wash out the bladder and "double
emptying" to empty it: emptying the bladder once; waiting a little,
standing up and sitting down again to empty the bladder a second
time. Cranberry juice is known to work by altering the acidity of the
urine, providing a less favourable environment for bacterial
multiplication. Intercourse may facilitate the entry of bacteria,
probably by friction of the penis on the wall of the urethra. Use of a
lubricant before entry and emptying the bladder immediately after
intercourse may help by flushing out the bacteria from the urethra.

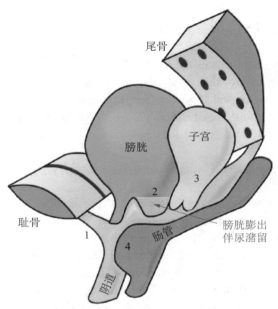

图 5-1 膀胱膨出与尿潴留 位点 2 膀胱膨出,向下形成一个囊性结构,阻碍尿液排空。随着时间迁延,尿液残留引起的感染会进展为慢性膀胱炎

　　在绝经后妇女中,防治慢性膀胱炎的第一道防线是阴道局部应用雌激素片剂或乳膏,开始每天 1 次,共 2 周;以后改为每周 3 次用药。雌激素能恢复阴道和尿道周围的海绵状结构。以这种方式给予的雌激素,主要作用于局部,不会引起乳腺癌。我们建议应有足量的尿液冲洗膀胱,并以"二次排尿"的方法排空膀胱,即嘱患者先排尿一次,等待片刻,起立后重新坐下再排尿一次。众所周知,蔓越莓汁能够改变尿液的酸度,造成不利于细菌繁殖的环境。性交会促进细菌的入侵,原因可能是阴茎对尿道壁的摩擦。在阴茎进入前使用润滑剂和在性交后立即排空膀胱有助于将细菌冲洗出尿道。

What Else May Cause Recurrent Cystitis?

Anything which irritates the inside of the bladder, such as a polyp (a non-cancerous growth), a bladder stone, or penetration of a plastic mesh after a surgical procedure for incontinence can cause recurrent cystitis. Inserting a cystoscope (a type of thin telescope) into the bladder is the best method for diagnosing such a problem.

What Else May Cause Abnormal Emptying?

Anything which interrupts the messages from the brain may cause this problem. One cause which is often stated is diabetes. However, we have found that many patients labelled as having "diabetic neuropathy" (damage to bladder nerves caused by diabetes) in fact had damaged ligaments in the back part of the vagina which prevented the opening muscles from working properly. Such patients had accompanying symptoms such as nocturia, urgency and pelvic pain, which indicated a problem in the back ligaments.

A Cystocele with Abnormal Emptying

Mrs VA was 53 years old with 4 teenage children. She gave this story.

"Every time I stand, a "squashy thing" comes out of the vagina. It is so uncomfortable. I have to sit in a funny position when I drive. I can't empty my bladder properly. I get 5 − 6 bladder infections a year. I am always in and out of the GP's office. My husband didn't like the "squashy thing" when we had sex, so he came with me to ask the GP what we could do about it. She suggested a pessary but we didn't like that idea much as we were still sexually active. The GP sent me off for a bladder repair. This was two years ago. The "squashy thing" came down again a few months after the operation. The GP tried a pessary this time round

还有什么会引起复发性膀胱炎？

任何刺激膀胱内壁的因素，例如息肉（非癌性生长的）、膀胱结石或尿失禁术后穿透入膀胱的合成材料，都可能引起复发性膀胱炎。膀胱镜（一种细的内窥镜）进入膀胱检查是诊断复发性膀胱炎的最佳方法。

还有什么可能引起排空异常？

任何干扰大脑信息传递的情况，都可能导致排空异常，其中最常见的是糖尿病。然而，我们发现许多"糖尿病神经性病变"（糖尿病引起的膀胱神经损伤）的患者，实际上已经存在阴道后部韧带的损伤，韧带损伤使膀胱逼尿肌不能正常工作。这些患者伴有的夜尿、尿急和盆腔疼痛等症状，都表明后部韧带出现了问题。

一例膀胱膨出伴有排空异常的患者

VA 太太，53 岁，有 4 个十几岁的孩子。她叙述了下面的故事。

"每一次我站起来，都会有一个"湿软的东西"从阴道里掉出来，很难受。开车的时候，我的坐姿很奇怪。我不能正常排空膀胱，每年有 5～6 次膀胱感染，频繁光顾于家庭医生的诊所。我的丈夫在和我同房时不喜欢这个"湿软的东西"，所以他和我一起去咨询家庭医生，我们该如何处理。医生建议我使用子宫托，我们不喜欢这个方案，因为我们的性生活还很频繁。两年前，家庭医生将我转诊去做了阴道前壁修补术。术后几个月，这

but it kept falling out. She said my vagina was short from the operation and that was why the pessary fell out. I went to see another surgeon. He said he would need to remove more vagina as part of the surgery. He said there was about a 60% chance that the operation would fail because the tissues were so poor".

We found that the vaginal tissue covering the cystocele was very thin and her vagina was a little short, all a result of the previous surgery. Clearly, no further tissue could be removed. A TFS operation which requires only an overnight stay was performed to support the prolapsed bladder without excision of vaginal tissue. The TFS is a relatively new method which inserts thin horizontal segments of tape to support the front wall of vagina like ceiling joists. No vaginal tissue is ever cut away. When reviewed at 12 months, the cystocele had disappeared and there were no further episodes of infection or abnormal emptying.

Severe Wetting on Getting Out of Bed in the Morning Caused by Excessive Scarring from Multiple Surgeries—a Hitherto Unrec-ognised Problem

Excessive scarring in the vagina from previous surgery, "tethered vagina", is a serious but not well recognized condition. Its defining symptom is sudden massive urine loss immediately on getting out of bed in the morning.

Mrs EM, 68 years old, was referred to our clinic with a history of worsening incontinence over the past 2 years. She had had 4 previous operations for prolapse and incontinence some years earlier. She volunteered the cardinal symptom of this condition.

"My bladder empties uncontrollably immediately my foot touches the floor on getting out of bed in the morning. I also lose urine on standing up from a chair or bending down. I just can't risk going out any more, not even to meet my friends. My husband has to do the shopping."

个"湿软的东西"又掉落下来了。家庭医生再次尝试戴子宫托，
但它经常掉出来。她说我的阴道在阴道前壁修补术后变短了，
这就是子宫托脱落的原因。我去看了另一个外科医生。他跟我
说需要切除更多的阴道壁，因为这是手术的一部分，但由于组织
过于薄弱，手术有60％的概率失败。"

我们检查发现，先前的手术使覆盖在膨出膀胱上的阴道壁
组织变得非常薄，阴道也有些短。显然，已经无法再切除更多的
组织。TFS手术可支撑脱垂的膀胱，只需住院一晚，不用切除
阴道壁组织。TFS手术是一种新的手术方法，即从水平方向置
入细条状吊带，像吊顶龙骨一样支撑阴道前壁，而不用切除阴道
壁组织。术后第12个月复查时，VA太太的膀胱膨出消失了，
再没有发生膀胱感染或排空异常。

多次手术所致阴道壁过度瘢痕化，引起严重的晨起尿失禁——一个至今未被认识的问题

既往手术造成的阴道过度瘢痕化，称为"阴道束缚症"，是一
种严重但尚未得到公认的疾病，其典型症状是早晨起床时突然
大量漏尿。

EM太太，68岁，转诊到我们诊所时，有日益加重的尿失禁
2年。在过去的几年间，她曾因脱垂和尿失禁进行过4次手术。
她有阴道束缚症的主要症状。

"早上起床时，我的脚一碰到地板，就控制不住地漏尿。从
椅子上站起来或弯腰时也会漏尿。我再也不能冒险出门，甚至
不能去约见我的朋友，购物只能由丈夫代劳。"

She denied any significant urine loss on coughing and this was confirmed on examination. The large amount of urine measured with the 24 hour pad test validated the seriousness of this lady's problem. There was very little movement of her bladder neck during straining with ultrasound testing, consistent with the thick scarring we observed in the front part of her vagina. A skin graft placed in this area restored elasticity and vastly improved her incontinence.

Comment 1 on excessive scarring of the vagina from previous surgeries

This is still not a well-recognized condition and it is invariably caused by excessive scarring from previous surgeries. This condition was not previously recognized as originating from a scarred vagina. It was thought to originate from the bladder itself and was (still is, by many!) treated with drugs, which, of course, cannot succeed, as the problem is that scarring causes loss of elasticity in the vagina. The skin graft restored elasticity and cured the patient. This is one of the many so-called " incurable " conditions which can be addressed by applying the Integral System.

Comment 2 on excessive scarring and tissue deficit of the vagina

In 2011 Professor Petros visited the Hamlin Hospital in Addis Ababa Ethiopia to work on the problem of severe incontinence following successful fistula repair which occurs in 25% of cases. It was found that many of these problems were caused by tissue deficit and scarring in the vagina, similar to Mrs EM and so were potentially curable with a skin graft at the time of fistula repair, or afterwards. These are preliminary findings, but they offer hope for many thousands of such women.

她否认咳嗽时有明显的漏尿，这也在检查中得到了证实。通过 24 小时尿垫试验发现大量漏尿，证明这位太太的问题非常严重。超声检查提示，她在做向下屏气动作时，膀胱颈的移动度很小，这与我们观察到阴道前壁有增厚的瘢痕一致。瘢痕部位的皮瓣移植恢复了阴道前壁的弹性，极大地改善了她的尿失禁症状。

点评 1　既往手术造成的阴道壁过度瘢痕化

由既往手术造成的过度瘢痕化，导致阴道束缚，并未得到公认。此前没有人认为尿失禁是由于瘢痕化的阴道引起。人们认为它起源于膀胱本身（至今仍有很多人这样认为！），并用药物治疗。事实上，这种治疗是无效的，因为问题的根源在于瘢痕导致阴道组织失去弹性。皮瓣移植恢复了阴道的弹性，治愈了患者。这是应用"整体理论系统"解决的诸多所谓"不治之症"之一。

点评 2　阴道过度瘢痕化和组织缺损

2011 年，Petros 教授访问了埃塞俄比亚首都亚的斯亚贝巴（Addis Ababa）的 Hamlin 医院，着手解决膀胱瘘修补成功后，25% 的患者出现严重尿失禁的问题。研究发现，这种情况多数是由阴道组织缺损和瘢痕造成的，和 EM 太太的情况类似，可在膀胱瘘修补的同时或修补后应用皮瓣移植治愈。虽然这只是初步的发现，但也为成千上万罹患阴道束缚症的女性带来了希望。

（上海交通大学医学院附属第六人民医院妇产科，黄程胜　译，吴氢凯　校）

CHAPTER 6 Is This Your Problem?

—Back ligament damage

The back ligaments when damaged can cause prolapse of the uterus, which descends down the vagina as a firm "lump". If the tissue damage is in the middle or lower part of the vagina, the patient may complain of a soft "lump" called a rectocele. However, not all prolapses have symptoms.

The Main Symptoms of Back Ligament Looseness

These are urgency, getting up at night to pass urine more than twice 'nocturia', low dragging pain in the lower abdomen, pain on deep penetration with intercourse, "vulvodynia", (hypersensitivity or "burning" at the entrance of vagina), inability to empty the bladder properly, and sometimes faecal incontinence. However, quite major symptoms can occur with only minimal prolapse of the uterus.

Nocturia, Urgency, Abnormal Emptying and Pelvic Pain Caused by Looseness in the Back Ligaments

Mrs LM was 53 years old. She stated,

"I get up 4 - 5 times a night. I find this very tiring as I have to work next day. I have a dragging pain on the right side which can be quite distracting by the end of the day. I am always going to the toilet at work. My urine dribbles away after I stand up and I often wet the toilet seat. I have problems with bladder infections. My first GP did a whole lot of x-rays, a CT scan, blood tests for the pain. I went to a gynaecologist who put a tube into my tummy and found nothing. She said that she couldn't find anything wrong and she sent me to a psychiatrist, because she thought the pain

第六章　您有这样的问题吗?
——后部韧带损伤

后部韧带受损时会引起子宫脱垂(prolapse of the uterus),子宫像一个"硬块"沿着阴道下降。当阴道中部或下部组织损伤时,患者可能描述为"软块",即"直肠膨出(rectocele)"。但是,并非所有脱垂都会有症状。

后部韧带松弛的主要症状

症状为:尿急,每晚起床排尿两次以上(夜尿症),下腹部牵拉痛,深部性交痛,"外阴痛"(阴道口过度敏感或有"灼烧感"),无法完全排空膀胱和时有发生的粪失禁。

但即便最轻微的子宫脱垂,也可能出现相当严重的症状。

后部韧带松弛引起的夜尿、尿急、膀胱排空异常和盆腔疼痛

LM 太太,53 岁。她说道:

"我每晚得起床 4～5 次。这让我感到很累,因为第二天我还得工作。右侧(腹部)会感到牵拉样的疼痛,每到晚上尤为明显。我经常在工作的时候上厕所,站起来时尿液就会流出来,常常弄湿马桶座圈。我有膀胱感染。为了寻找病因,我的第一位家庭医生给我做了好多 X 线片、CT 扫描以及血液检查。我去

was in my head. He said there was nothing wrong psychologically. I saw many GPs and several specialists about the bladder. They gave me tablets to stop the bladder from working so frequently but these made my emptying worse and they gave me a dry mouth as well, so I had to stop taking them. They said they couldn't do anything else for me. One even said it might all be in my head. Mostly they said I had to learn to put up with these symptoms, because they were incurable. I came here because I felt a lump coming out. "

Mrs LM had symptoms typical of looseness in the back ligaments. When we examined her, we noted that her uterus was protruding outside the vagina. We inserted a TFS "minisling" to repair her back ligaments. This repaired the prolapse and tightened the vaginal membrane. It was minimal surgery performed entirely from the vagina. Mrs LM required only an overnight stay in hospital and she returned to work in 7 days. When reviewed at 9 months, she was getting up only once per night to empty her bladder. She said that her low abdominal pain was still present but was 90% better and it rarely bothered her now. Her bladder emptying also was not entirely cured but had improved significantly and she had not had any bladder infections since the operation.

Characteristics of pelvic pain caused by back ligament looseness

- Almost invariably occurs with other symptoms, specifically urgency, nocturia, abnormal emptying.
- Low abdominal 'dragging' pain, usually one side, often right-sided.
- Low sacral pain (pain near the tailbone)—present in 50% of cases.
- Pain on deep penetration with intercourse.
- Low abdominal ache the next day after intercourse.
- Pain worsens during the day and is relieved by lying down.
- Pain is reproduced on pressing the cervix or the back wall of the

看妇科，医生做了腹腔镜检查，但一无所获。她说她不知道问题出在哪里，让我去看精神科，因为她觉得疼痛来自大脑的臆想。但精神科医生却认为我心理上没有问题。我看了许多家庭医生和泌尿科专家，他们让我服用抑制尿频的药，但服药后膀胱更难排空了。这些药还有口干的不良反应，因此我不得不停止服药。医生说他们也束手无策，甚至有人说这可能都是我臆想出来的。多数人认为我的疼痛无法治疗，所以我只能试图去适应它。而我到这个诊所来，是因为我感觉到有块东西脱出来了。"

LM 太太有典型的后部韧带松弛症状。检查时，我们发现子宫脱出于阴道外。我们手术置入 TFS"迷你吊带（minisling）"来修复她的后部韧带，这样可以修复脱垂并拉紧阴道吊床。这种微创手术完全经阴道完成。LM 太太术后次日就出院了，7 天就重返工作岗位。在 9 个月的随访期内，她每晚只需起床一次排尿。她说下腹痛仍然存在，但已经缓解了 90%，现在基本上不会困扰她了。她的膀胱排空问题并未完全治愈，但有明显改善，术后膀胱感染也再未发生过。

后部韧带松弛引起的盆腔疼痛的特征

- 几乎总是伴随其他症状，尤其是尿急、夜尿、膀胱排空异常。
- 下腹部"牵拉样"疼痛，通常为单侧，右侧居多。
- 尾骶部疼痛（近尾骨处疼痛）——存在于 50% 的病例中。
- 性交时的深部触痛。
- 性交后第二天出现下腹痛。
- 白天疼痛加剧，平卧时缓解。

vagina if a patient has had a hysterectomy.

- Tiredness-worsening during the day.
- Irritability-worsening during the day.

Pain During Intercourse and Bowel Problems Caused by Back Ligament Looseness

Mrs RM was a hard-working 47 year old mother of 2 who worked in a Nursing Home. She stated,

"I always have urgency to empty my bowel but I am also frequently constipated. I get up 3 – 4 times a night to pass urine. I have problems emptying my bladder. My worst problem is that I can't have sex any more. Almost every time I have intercourse, my bowels open. It is so horrible. My husband is very understanding but I am sure he is as distressed as I am. I always have pain on deep penetration. Often I have a dragging pain low down on my right side which seems to get worse by the end of the day".

She had 2 teenage sons and helped her husband in his business in her spare time. At one stage she had sought medical advice but was told she could not be helped. After confiding her problem to a close a friend who had been to the clinic, she was persuaded to make an appointment. Many patients came to the clinic in this way.

Her symptoms of nocturia and abnormal emptying indicated damage in the back ligaments. When we examined her, there was very minimal prolapse. As Mrs RM's problems were complex, we recommended that we repair only the back ligaments and then we would reassess her. We advised her that she could expect a cure rate of 80% for some of her symptoms. As for the urge to empty her bowel and constipation, these could be due to many other causes, so we were reluctant to predict a cure for these symptoms.

We inserted a TFS "minisling" to repair the back ligaments. Mrs RM was discharged the next day with very little pain and she went back to work the following week. She attended with her husband for the post-operative visit. She was smiling and confident. She

- 按压宫颈,或按压子宫切除术后患者的阴道后壁会再现疼痛。
- 疲劳:白天加重。
- 烦躁:白天加重。

后部韧带松弛引起的性交痛和肠道问题

RM 太太,47 岁,是有两个孩子的勤劳母亲,在养老院工作。她说:

"我总感觉急迫地想解大便,但也经常便秘。我每晚起床小便 3~4 次,也难以排空膀胱。最糟糕的是,我再也无法有性生活了,几乎在每次性交的同时,大便就会排出来,这太可怕了。我丈夫非常理解我,但我知道他和我一样痛苦。我经常感到深部的触痛,以及右下腹牵拉样疼痛,夜间尤其明显。"

她有两个十几岁的儿子,业余时间帮助丈夫打理生意。有段时间她曾四处求医,但都被告知无能为力。后来,她将自己的烦恼告诉了一位曾经来过我们诊所的闺蜜,对方劝她预约来试一试。许多患者都是通过这样的方式来到我们诊所的。

夜尿和膀胱排空异常表明患者的后部韧带有损伤。查体时,我们发现她的脱垂程度很轻。由于 RM 太太的问题很复杂,我们建议只单纯修复后部韧带,再对她重新评估。我们告知她,部分症状可能会得到 80% 的缓解,而大便急迫和便秘的问题可能是由于其他原因引起的,因此我们暂不去估计它们的疗效。我们通过手术置入 TFS"迷你吊带"来修复后部韧带。RM太太术后几乎没有痛苦,次日出院,一周后便恢复了工作。后来她和丈夫一起来术后随访,她面带微笑并且充满自信。她无法抑制自己的激动:"我痊愈了,所有症状都消失了。"在私

could not contain her excitement and said to the secretary, "I'm cured. It's all gone". In the privacy of the consulting room, she reported cure of all her bowel symptoms and a major improvement in her other symptoms. Her husband said, "you don't know what a burden has been lifted from our lives". Mrs RM remained cured at last review 4 years later.

Mrs RM is a good example of the passive "Conspiracy of Silence", a reticence to discuss this condition, even between man and wife. Without input from her friend, Mrs RM is unlikely to have sought assistance. Even with patients who do come to see us, faecal soiling is rarely volunteered in a face to face situation, another "Conspiracy of Silence", this time, even with her doctor.

This is why it is important for patients to take the questionnaire (a series of printed questions) home and to answer the questions in their own time. It is so much easier to write it down, than to say it as it becomes almost anonymous.

Comment on losing faeces during intercourse

This patient was a challenge to us, as some of her symptoms were not the typical symptoms seen with damage in the back ligaments. We had encountered women opening their bladder during intercourse before but never their bowel. In such cases, we simply repair the ligaments which we can see have been damaged, following the guiding principle of this method, "repair the structure, and you will restore the function".

Comment on pain with intercourse

The back ligaments form an important support for the pain nerves contained inside them. Earlier we discussed how a loose ligament will not support nerve fibres. As the penis thrusts into the back part of the vagina, it will cause pain if it stretches the unsupported nerve fibres.

密的诊室里,她表示所有肠道症状都治愈了,其他症状也得到了明显改善。她的丈夫说:"你不知道这给我们的生活减轻了多少负担。"RM 太太在 4 年的随访期结束前,仍然保持着良好的疗效。

RM 太太是被动"缄默的密约"的范例,即使夫妻之间,彼此也不愿意讨论这种尴尬问题。如果没有闺蜜的开导,RM 太太也不大可能会寻求帮助。部分患者即便来找我们,在面对面的场合里也难以主动谈及大便漏出的问题,这是另一种"缄默的密约",即使对医生也难以启齿。这就是为什么让患者把问卷(一串打印出来的问题)带回家,并在私人时间内填写是如此重要的原因。由于多数问卷是匿名填写的,因此写下来比说出来要容易得多。

对性交时粪失禁的点评

这位患者对于我们是一个挑战,因为她的某些症状不是后部韧带损伤的典型表现。我们曾经遇到过性交时漏尿的妇女,但粪失禁是第一次见到。对于这位患者,我们只是按指导原则修复了已知损伤的韧带,即"修复解剖,可重建功能"。

对性交痛的点评

后部韧带对穿行其中的痛觉神经构成了重要的支持。先前我们讨论了由于韧带松弛,导致神经纤维失去支持。当阴茎触碰阴道后壁时,牵扯了缺少支撑的神经纤维,会引起疼痛。

Severe Pelvic Pain Caused by Back ligament looseness

Mrs D was a 34 year old science teacher from London, UK. She attended with severe pain in the right side of her abdomen. Some years previously, she had attended a London hospital where the Professor had created an international reputation using psychological tests to prove that such pain was psychological in origin.

Mrs D had read widely on the subject of pain. Her facial expression indicated a person who was guarded. Her face lit up after she answered positively to the following questions because she suddenly became aware that we knew what her problem was.

- Do you have pain on deep penetration with intercourse?
- Do you get up more than twice per night to pass urine?
- Do you have problems emptying your bladder?
- Do you have urgency?

Positive answers to at least some symptoms other than pain are required before we can predict that the pain is caused by damage to the back ligaments. There are, after all, many other causes of chronic pelvic pain in the 30 plus age group, for example, endometriosis, infection in the Fallopian tubes, problems with large intestine, to name just a few.

This is what she said one week after her pain was cured by a small operation which tightened her back ligaments.

"I was almost suicidal after interminable attacks of pain on my right side. It has now been a week since the operation and I feel like a rabbit that has been released from a trap. My mind keeps scanning up and down my body searching for the pain which for so long has been my centre and focus."

The operation was simple, and it was performed entirely under local anaesthesia. A 3 cm incision was made in the vagina behind the cervix. Two sutures were inserted to tighten the ligaments.

后部韧带松弛引起的严重盆腔疼痛

D 太太,34 岁,英国伦敦的科学老师。她右侧腹痛相当严重。数年前,她曾在伦敦的一家医院接受治疗,该院的教授在国际上享有盛誉,因为他用心理学测试来证明这类疼痛是心因性的。

D 太太对于疼痛的话题已经做足了功课。起初她的面部表情是戒备的。在对以下问题做出肯定的回答后,她的脸泛红了,因为她突然意识到我们知道她的症结所在。

- 您在性交时是否有深部触痛?
- 您每晚起床两次以上来排尿吗?
- 您排空膀胱有困难吗?
- 您有尿急吗?

在我们可以推测疼痛是由后部韧带损伤引起之前,至少需要对疼痛以外的其他症状做出肯定的回答。毕竟,在 30 岁以上的人群中,还有许多其他原因能引起慢性盆腔疼痛,如子宫内膜异位症、输卵管炎、结肠病变等。

我们通过一个小手术收紧了她的后部韧带,一周后,疼痛得到了缓解,她如是说:

"无休止的右侧腹痛,几乎让我想要自杀。现在手术已过去一周,我感觉自己就像是一只从牢笼里被释放出来的兔子。潜意识里仍上下搜寻那个长期以来占据我生活重心的痛点,但它消失了!

手术很简单,完全可在局部麻醉下进行。我们在宫颈后方的阴道,做一个 3 cm 的切口,缝合韧带 2 针,并打结收紧。

Comment on understanding the causation of dragging lower abdominal pain

Unfortunately, this condition, severe pelvic pain caused by loose back ligaments, is still not well recognized by the majority of gynaecologists and yet the cure is so simple.
Postscript Mrs D. wrote to the Professor in England and told him her story. She sent him some published scientific articles which described cure of urgency, frequency, nocturia, and pelvic pain. He could not understand the relationship between all these symptoms, or that her pelvic pain could be cured in such a simple way. He wrote back and said "but these articles are about bladder problems". He just did not understand the ramifications of the "Integral System" which our clinic was applying. It is difficult even for the most learned person to associate lower abdominal pain with apparently unrelated symptoms such as urge and frequency which are thought to arise from the bladder.

Vulvodynia-Pain and Burning at the Entrance to the Vagina ("Vulvodynia") Caused by Back Ligament Looseness

• There are many causes of "vulvodynia", including skin conditions. The type we are describing is associated with low abdominal pain, urgency, nocturia and abnormal bladder emptying.
Mrs P was 49 years old. She had chronic pelvic pain and she requested referral to the clinic because she had heard that we were achieving good results in patients with pelvic pain. Her General Practitioner, an empathetic and caring man, rang the doctor before she arrived and asked that we "handle her very carefully" as she was severely disturbed psychologically, that this was the reason for her pain and there was nothing anyone could do for her. The first impression we had of this lady did indeed fit the description of her GP. Her face was contorted, she spoke rapidly and with

对找到下腹牵拉痛病因的点评

遗憾的是,关于严重的盆腔疼痛往往由后部韧带松弛引起,并且治愈方法是如此简单的观点,仍未被大多数妇科医生所接受。

附言　D太太给英国的教授写信讲述了她的故事,并寄给他一些描述如何治疗尿急、尿频、夜尿和盆腔疼痛的文献。但那位教授依然无法理解这些症状之间的关系,也无法理解竟用如此简单的手术就治愈了她的盆腔疼痛。他回信说:"可这些文章都是关于膀胱问题的。"他只是尚未理解我们诊所正在应用的"整体理论系统"的效力。看来即使是最有学问的人,也很难将下腹痛与似乎无关的症状(如被认为来自膀胱的尿频和尿急症状)联系起来。

外阴痛——后部韧带松弛引起的阴道口疼痛和烧灼感("外阴痛")

- "外阴痛"有很多病因,包括皮肤病变。我们所描述的类型与下腹痛、尿急、夜尿症和膀胱排空异常有关。

P太太,49岁,患有慢性盆腔痛。她听闻我们治疗盆腔疼痛有很好的疗效,因此要求转诊至我们诊所。她的家庭医生是一个充满同情心和体贴的人,在她到来前就致电要求我们"非常小心地接待她",因为她的心理遭受着严重的困扰,这是她痛苦的原因,再做什么都无济于事了。我们对这位女士的第一印象确实符合家庭医生的描述。她的面部是扭曲的,语速快且有明显的焦虑。多年来,她因为疼痛而拜访了许多专家。她接受

obvious anxiety. She had visited many specialists over the years for her pain. She had undergone several diagnostic laparoscopies (a type of telescope inserted into the abdomen to view the uterus and ovaries), even a hysterectomy and had attended a pain clinic. None of these treatments had helped her pain. The consensus from other specialists as reported to the GP was that her problem was psychological. Her replies to the questionnaire gave the first hint that this woman may have a physical cause for her problem, damage to her back ligaments. She woke 6 times per night to empty her bladder (nocturia), wore pads continually as she wet 6 times per day (urge incontinence) and had difficulties emptying her bladder. She also had faecal incontinence. We asked her if she had told her GP about her bladder and bowel problems. She said she had only consulted him about the burning pain around her vagina and anus. She said that her vagina was so tender that she couldn't have sexual intercourse and sometimes had problems sitting. Examination revealed a prolapse of the back part of her vagina. The entrance to the vagina was hypersensitive-she recoiled when gently tested with a cotton bud, the classical test for "vulvodynia" (pain at the entrance of the vagina).

We did not claim that we could cure this lady's pain, as there are many other causes for pelvic pain. Nevertheless, it was explained that her vaginal prolapse needed to be fixed and that there was a strong possibility that some of her symptoms would also improve with a sling inserted into the back part of her vagina, a fairly minor day-care procedure.

The first thing we noticed at the 6 week post-operative visit was the absence of tension in her face. She was smiling and calm. Her pain was gone, as was her urgency and faecal incontinence. Her nocturia had reduced to 2 per night and her bladder emptying was "60% improved".

Like the case of Mrs D, this lady's problem raises many issues about the attitudes of doctors, patients, even modern medicine itself. Many doctors, including this lady's General Practitioner, were not aware that this type of pelvic pain is associated with loose ligaments. Because of the scientific nature of medicine, if an obvious cause cannot be found, the doctor seeks another cause, usually "psychological".

了几次诊断性腹腔镜检查（一种置入腹腔的检查镜，用于观察子宫和卵巢），甚至进行了子宫切除术，并去过一家疼痛诊所。但这些疗法都没能减轻她的痛苦。其他专家都不约而同地向家庭医生报告说她的问题来自心理。但问卷调查的结果初步提示，这位女士的疼痛可能由躯体疾病引起，即后部韧带损伤。她每晚有6次醒来排尿（夜尿症），在持续使用护垫的情况下，每天有6次浸湿护垫（急迫性尿失禁），并且有膀胱排空困难和大便失禁。我们问她是否告诉过家庭医生膀胱和肠道的情况，她说她只咨询过阴道口和肛周灼痛。她说自己的阴道太脆弱以至于无法进行性交，有时坐着也会有不适。我们为她查体时发现她有阴道后壁脱垂，以及阴道口过度敏感——当用棉签轻轻触碰时，她会向后躲避，这是"外阴痛"（阴道口疼痛）的经典试验。

我们并未声称可以治愈这位女士的疼痛，因为盆腔疼痛还有许多其他原因。尽管如此，我们仍向她解释：阴道脱垂需要修复。我们把吊带置入阴道后壁后，某些症状很可能会改善，而这是一个相当小的日间手术。

术后6周复诊时，我们注意到的第一件事是她脸上的紧张消失了。她面带微笑而且平静，疼痛、尿急和大便失禁都消失了。夜尿频率已减少至每晚2次，膀胱排空情况也"改善了60%"。

正如D太太的病例，这位女士的难题引发了许多关于医生、患者甚至现代医学本身对类似病情看法的争议。许多医生，包括这位女士的家庭医生，都没有意识到这种盆腔疼痛与韧带松弛有关。由于医学的科学性质，如果无法找到明显的病因，医生会寻找其他原因来解释，通常会归结为"心理"因素。

将心理障碍作为疾病的根源，其概念可以追溯到西格蒙

The concept of psychological disturbance as the root cause of a medical condition can be traced back to Sigmund Freud himself. However, any type of chronic pain is sufficient to unsettle even the most rational person and such patients do become psychologically disturbed, often severely, as we saw in several of the histories. According to our experience, it is the pain which causes the psychological disturbance, not the other way round. Whether it be Freud's influence, or exhaustion of all known physical causes * , attributing these difficult problems to a psychological cause is an important contributor to the "Conspiracy of Silence". No woman wishes to be labelled a "nut case". As soon as a psychological causation has been hinted at, she becomes silent. She remains so for all subsequent medical consultations, another contributor to the " Conspiracy of Silence ". Our experience is that modern women are far too busy to complain about symptoms they do not have.

Comment on Whether it be Freud's influence, or exhaustion of all known physical causes···.. There is another possibility, a new discovery which can address these so-called "incurable" problems of incontinence and pelvic pain. That is why we wrote this book, to inform women that a cure for these conditions already exists and to use this knowledge, especially the patient histories, to empower them when they choose to seek treatment for such problems.

Characteristics of ' Vulvodynia '

Vulvodynia which has no apparent local cause (such as a skin condition) is often expressed by a burning pain over the entrance of the vagina and anus with extreme sensitivity on touching, often associated with dragging lower abdominal pain and sometimes, painful bladder conditions.

Comment on causes of vulvodynia

We do not claim that all vulvodynia patients have this cause. However,

德·弗洛伊德(Sigmund Freud)本人。但是,任何类型的慢性疼痛都足以使最理性的人不安,而且正如我们在既往的各个病例中所见,此类患者的确会受到心理上的困扰,而且通常是严重的困扰。但根据我们的经验,恰恰相反,是疼痛造成了心理障碍。无论是受弗洛伊德的影响,还是将所有已知躯体因素所造成的"精疲力竭",把这些难题归因于心理因素都是"缄默的密约"的重要原因。没有女人愿意被贴上"疯子"的标签。一旦被暗示为心理因素,她就会保持沉默。在随后的所有医疗咨询中,她会习惯性如此,使自身成为"缄默的密约"的另一推动者。就我们的经验来看,现代女性已经太过繁忙,根本无暇抱怨她们所没有的症状。

对"无论是受弗洛伊德的影响,还是将所有已知躯体因素造成的精疲力竭……"的点评,还有另一种可能性:一项新发现可以解决这些所谓的"无法治愈"的尿失禁和盆腔疼痛问题。这也是我们撰写本书的目的,是要告知广大妇女这类疾病是可治愈的,并利用这些知识,尤其是患者的亲身经历,她们可以自主把握命运。

"外阴痛"的特征

没有明显局部原因(如皮肤状况)的外阴痛常表现为阴道和肛门入口的烧灼样疼痛,它对触碰极为敏感,通常与下腹部牵拉样疼痛有关,有时还伴有膀胱疼痛症。

对外阴痛的点评

我们并不是说所有的外阴痛都由此所致。但如果将后部韧

if other symptoms of back ligament looseness such as nocturia, abnormal bladder emptying, and urgency are grouped with the vulvodynia, there is a strong possibility that this pain can be improved in many patients with a posterior sling for repair of the back ligaments.

Tampon test—A simple test to see if the back ligaments

We have found that a large tampon inserted into the back part of the vagina as a test can often instantaneously relieve the sensitivity and pain in the vulva. Generally such women also have other back ligament symptoms.

Pelvic Pain Commencing Soon After the First Period Caused by Back Ligament Looseness

Miss PN was 23 years old. She complained of severe pelvic pain which began some months after her first period at the age of 15. The pain was worse at period time. She had already undergone two laparoscopies where nothing was found. The doctor thought her problem was psychological and she had been referred to a psychiatrist. She came to the clinic with her mother, who was certain that her daughter was not only psychologically normal but there was some physical reason for the pain.

On assessment, it was clear to us that Miss PN had looseness in her back ligaments dating from birth, a looseness exacerbated by hormones from her periods. The ligaments were just not strong enough. She had symptoms of urge and nocturia. These symptoms were all worse at period time. We explained that at period time, the brain secretes a hormone which relaxes the collagen fibres in the cervix sufficiently for the menstrual blood to exit the uterus. This relaxation also loosens the ligaments which are attached to the uterus, causing her symptoms of pain and urge to worsen.

Miss PN did not respond to the pelvic floor exercises which were prescribed prior to surgery but had a very good result when the back ligaments were surgically tightened with a minor day-care

带松弛的其他症状（如夜尿、膀胱排空困难和尿急）与外阴痛结合在一起，应用吊带修补后部韧带后，很可能使这种疼痛得到缓解。

卫生棉条试验——一个简单的测试，看看后部韧带是否出现了问题

我们发现，将大号卫生棉条置入阴道后部，外阴敏感和疼痛常可立即缓解。通常这类女性还有其他后部韧带的症状。

后部韧带松弛引起的初潮后盆腔疼痛

PN 小姐，23 岁，15 岁初潮的几个月后，她便开始感觉到严重的盆腔疼痛。疼痛在经期加剧。目前她已经接受了两次腹腔镜检查，均未发现异常。医生认为她有心理上的问题，便将她转诊给精神科医生。她和母亲一起来到我们的诊所，母亲坚信女儿在心理上是正常的，认为是某种躯体的病因导致了疼痛。

经评估，我们发现，PN 小姐有与生俱来的后部韧带松弛，这种松弛情况随月经周期激素的变化而加剧。由于韧带不够坚强，导致尿急和夜尿的症状，且在经期加剧。我们的解释是：在经期，大脑会分泌一种激素，使宫颈中的胶原纤维充分松弛，以便月经血排出子宫。这种作用也会使附着在子宫上的韧带松弛，导致疼痛和尿急症状加重。

手术前，先建议 PN 小姐施行盆底训练，但效果不明显。而缩短后部韧带的日间小手术取得了很好的成效。术中没有使用吊带，因此对她日后的生育能力毫无影响。

operation. No tapes were used and this did not affect her ability to have children in any way.

Hysterectomy for Lower Backache and Pelvic Pain Caused by Back Ligament Looseness

Mrs JMK developed chronic lower back pain and pain with intercourse after a difficult forceps delivery of her second child 50 years ago when she was 27 years old. The pain as described earlier was constant and debilitating. At age 35, a specialist gynaecologist advised hysterectomy. This caused a major emotional shock, as she wished to have more children. She was persuaded to proceed with the operation. The operation did not go so well initially. She needed a blood transfusion during the surgery. Because of continuing anaemia, she remained weak for another 6 months. Although the physical pain had improved, Mrs JMK was mentally traumatized by the hysterectomy for some time afterwards. By the time she was 65 years old, the chronic pelvic pain and lower backache had returned, along with urgency, nocturia and prolapse of the vagina and bladder. We attributed all this to age-related loss of collagen and weakening of the back ligaments, a long-term problem in many patients who have had hysterectomy. Ligament reconstruction cured the prolapse and greatly improved the symptoms.

Comment on hysterectomy   Removal of the uterus is a major operation. It is not always complication-free and may have long-term physical and psychological consequences for some women. Fortunately, minor treatments for uterine haemorrhage, for example, intrauterine devices which slowly leach progesterone-type hormones, are now available.

Abnormal Emptying and Chronic Bladder Infection Caused by Looseness in the Back Ligaments

Mrs KB, a 32 year old flight attendant had a long history of

用子宫切除术治疗因后部韧带松弛引起的下背部疼痛和盆腔疼痛

JMK 太太,在 50 年前(27 岁)生第二个孩子时因难产使用产钳助产,此后便出现了慢性下背部疼痛和性交痛。当时疼痛是持续的,并且使她感到虚弱。35 岁时,一名妇科医生建议她切除子宫。因为她希望有更多孩子,所以她在情感上难以接受,但最终她被说服了。手术一开始并不顺利,术中输了血。由于持续贫血,她在术后 6 个月都比较虚弱。尽管身体上的疼痛有所改善,但因为切除了子宫,她受到了精神上的创伤。到 65 岁时,慢性盆腔痛和下背痛又出现了,随之而来的还有尿急、夜尿症、阴道和膀胱脱垂。我们将所有这些症状归因于与年龄相关的胶原蛋白丢失和后部韧带减弱,这是许多子宫切除术后患者的远期问题。韧带重建可以治疗脱垂,并大大改善上述症状。

对子宫切除术的点评 子宫切除术是一个大手术,有时会出现并发症,可能对部分妇女造成长期的身心影响。幸运的是,现在有一些创伤小的方法可以治疗子宫出血,例如可以缓慢释放孕激素的宫内节育器。

后部韧带松弛引起的膀胱排空异常和慢性膀胱感染

KB 小姐,32 岁,空姐。她从十几岁开始,一直无法排空膀胱且有慢性膀胱感染。她是一个衣着精致、个性迷人的年轻女性。她来找我们是因为感染变得越来越频繁,影响到她在长途飞行中的工作。她的病情发展让她不得不考虑转行。我们的诊

inability to empty her bladder and chronic bladder infections, dating back to her teenage years. She was a well groomed young woman with an engaging personality. She came to us because the infections were becoming more frequent and they were affecting her ability to work on long flights. Her situation had reached a stage where she felt forced to consider leaving her profession. She was diagnosed as having congenitally weak back ligaments. She did not respond to our pelvic floor regime and she requested surgical reconstruction of the ligaments. We agreed, after having advised her that she may need a Caesarian Section if she fell pregnant, as any vaginal delivery could disrupt her operation. Her bladder returned to normal emptying immediately after the surgery and she reported no further bladder infections even after 10 years.

Comment on symptoms of bladder emptying difficulty

Typical symptoms are a slow stream, starting and stopping, dribbling on standing up after bladder emptying has been completed and a feeling that the bladder has not emptied. Often such patients have chronic urinary infections.

Comment on abnormal bladder emptying in the younger woman

Congenitally weak back ligaments must always be considered as a cause of abnormal bladder emptying in the younger woman as these women do not generally have a bulge in the front wall of the vagina (cystocele). Increased difficulty in emptying the bladder at period time in such women is highly suggestive that the cause is looseness in the back ligaments. Other symptoms such as pelvic pain, urgency and nocturia are frequently present and these may become worse during period time. Though not helpful with Mrs KB, good results in young women have been achieved at our clinic by encouraging such patients to " squat" instead of bending

断是：先天性后部韧带薄弱。盆底训练效果不佳，她要求进行韧带重建手术。我们告知她，术后若怀孕可能需要行剖宫产术，因为阴道分娩可能破坏手术效果。在征得她的同意后，我们进行了手术。手术后，她立刻能正常排空膀胱，直到 10 年后，她都没有患过膀胱感染。

对膀胱排空困难的点评

典型的症状是尿流缓慢、间断排尿、小便后起身时发生漏尿，感觉膀胱没有完全排空。这类患者经常患有慢性尿路感染。

对年轻女性膀胱排空异常的点评

先天性后部韧带薄弱通常是导致年轻女性膀胱排空异常的原因，她们往往在阴道前壁并没有凸起（膀胱膨出）。如果月经期膀胱排空更加困难，则高度提示是后部韧带松弛所致。其他症状，如盆腔痛、尿急和夜尿在月经期也很常见，并可能会加重。我们鼓励此类患者在日常生活中采取"下蹲动作"代替弯腰动作，工作中可坐在橡胶健身球上而不是椅子上。尽管这些建议对 KB 太太没有什么帮助，但已经在我们诊所的其他年轻女性中取得了良好的效果。这些训炼可加强盆底的肌肉和韧带。

as part of their daily routine and to sit on a rubber fitball at work instead of a chair. These exercises work by strengthening the pelvic muscles and ligaments.

An 87 Year Old Woman Unable to Pass Urine Requiring Catheterisation Caused by Back Ligament Looseness

There is a prevalence of this condition in nursing homes where many patients cannot pass urine and require indwelling catheters.
Mrs R was 87 years old, and weighed 90kg. She had had a hysterectomy 40 years earlier. For some years she needed to self-catheterize 3 – 4 times a day as she could not pass urine adequately. She had large residual volumes (the amount retained in the bladder after passing urine) and frequent urinary infections. On testing, we confirmed that she also had severe incontinence as she had a very large measured urine loss over a 24 hour period. She had major prolapse of the vagina, much like a glove turned inside out. We inserted a posterior sling and performed a rectocele repair. She passed urine immediately after the surgery. Her nocturia, previously 5 times per night, reduced to twice per night.

Comment on how age may cause ligament looseness and bladder emptying difficulties

The tissues of the vagina and its supporting ligaments may loosen considerably with age. The effect of this is that many older women, especially those in nursing homes, cannot empty their bladder and they require indwelling catheters (a catheter in the bladder all the time). These catheters are a major cause of chronic bladder infection as they introduce bacteria. We have returned many women to normal urination by reconstructing the back ligaments and tightening the neighbouring tissues.

一名87岁的妇女因后部韧带松弛无法排尿而留置导尿

这在养老院中是很普遍的情况,许多患者因排尿困难而需要留置导尿。

R太太,87岁,体重90千克。她40年前做了子宫切除手术。由于无法完全排净小便,几年来她每天进行3~4次自我导尿。她的残余尿量很大(排尿后残留在膀胱中的尿量),而且经常发生尿路感染。经检查,我们确定她患有严重的尿失禁,因为她每天24小时都有大量漏尿。她有严重的阴道脱垂,就像手套从里到外翻了个底朝天。我们通过手术置入了后部吊带,并进行了直肠膨出修补。她在术后立即可以自行排尿。术前夜尿每晚5次,术后减少到每晚2次。

对年龄增长可能引起韧带松弛和膀胱排空困难的点评

随着年龄的增长,阴道组织及其支持韧带可能会严重松弛。这导致许多老年女性,尤其是在养老院的老人无法排空膀胱,需要留置导尿(膀胱中持续置入导尿管)。这些导尿管可能带入细菌,成为慢性膀胱感染的主要原因。我们通过手术重建后部韧带,紧固周围组织,使许多妇女恢复了正常排尿功能。

会阴体修补治疗排便问题

VCD太太,46岁,有直肠膨出、大便失禁和排便困难的症状。她说:

Bowel Emptying Problems Cured by Repair of the Perineal Body

Mrs VCD, 46 years, presented with a rectocele, faecal incontinence and difficulty with emptying her bowel. She stated, *"Every time I need to open my bowels, I have to press my fingers into the back wall of my vagina so I can empty. I find the necessary hygiene after completion quite unpleasant."* In Mrs VCD's case, we found that the perineal bodies, the structures separating the vagina from the rectum had been pushed to each side. The vagina had been stretched very thinly and the bowel was bulging into it. That is why she had to press into the lower part of her vagina so she could open her bowels.

Because the perineal body sling was quite new at that time, she requested that her rectocele be repaired in the traditional way by forcibly suturing the perineal bodies together, a very painful operation. The rectocele and bowel evacuation difficulty were initially cured but recurred within 6 months, as did requirement to assist evacuation by pressing her fingers into the back wall of her vagina. On the second occasion, a TFS sling joined the perineal bodies to prevent the rectocele from protruding. This operation was far less painful than the traditional operation, where the perianal bodies were forcibly sutured together. She was now able to empty her bowel normally without a finger in her vagina. The rectocele remained cured at her 2 year review.

Urinary Urgency, Pelvic Pain and Nocturia Cured by Pelvic Floor Exercises

Miss B, a single 31 year old who had never been pregnant, gave this story.
"I began to experience symptoms of urgency, pelvic pain and nocturia at the age of 25, sufficiently to seek medical advice. I saw 8 different specialists. I was given drugs to stop the bladder

"每次需要排便时,我都必须用手指压迫阴道后壁才能排空大便。我觉得每次排便后的清洁工作让我很不愉快。"

在 VCD 太太的病例中,我们检查发现,会阴体这个将阴道与直肠隔开的结构被推到了两侧。阴道壁被膨出的直肠扩张得非常薄,直肠鼓进了阴道。因此,她必须用手指压迫阴道后壁下段才能促使肛门开放以排便。

因为当时会阴体吊带还是很新的技术,我们用传统的方法来修补直肠膨出,即将会阴体强行缝合在一起,患者术后会非常疼痛。最初,她的直肠膨出和排便困难已经治愈,但在 6 个月内复发,她依然需要手指按压阴道后壁来帮助排便。第二次手术时,我们采用 TFS 会阴体吊带来防止直肠膨出。与传统手术相比,这个手术痛苦要小得多,因为在传统手术中,肛周的组织被强行缝合在了一起。现在,她可以正常排便,无须再用手指压迫阴道排便。2 年后随访时,直肠仍未膨出。

盆底训练可以治疗尿急、盆腔疼痛和夜尿症

B 小姐,31 岁,单身女性,从未怀孕过。她讲述了下面的故事:

"我从 25 岁开始出现尿急、盆腔疼痛和夜尿的症状,四处求医问药。我看过 8 位不同的专家,他们给我药物以抑制膀胱收缩,我花了 10 000 美元在中草药上,但似乎都没有任何作用。"

最后,她通过中间人与我们诊所联系。她在海外工作,无法来诊所接受正式评估。我们建议她使用一个大的橡胶健身球代替椅子,并养成良好的保护盆底的习惯,例如尽可能下蹲(而不是弯腰),正确的站姿和盆底训练。结果是令人惊喜的——她

contracting. I spent $10,000 on Chinese herbal medicines. Nothing seemed to work".

Finally she contacted the clinic through an intermediary. She worked overseas and could not attend the clinic for a formal assessment. We advised her how to use a large rubber fitball as a substitute for a chair and to develop good pelvic floor habits such as squatting wherever possible (instead of bending), erect posture and exercise. The result was remarkable—virtually all her symptoms disappeared and she remained cured at last contact, 4 years later.

Comment on the non-surgical treatment of back ligament symptoms

A vast improvement in symptoms such as pelvic pain, urgency, abnormal emptying and nocturia has been achieved in many patients attending our clinic by the regime utilized by Miss B, in particular, substituting a "fitball" for a chair. This method is extremely time-efficient and is especially effective in the younger and middle-aged premenopausal woman.

Comment on the place of pelvic floor exercises in the treatment of incontinence today

The pelvic floor is as much part of the body as any other muscle group. It needs to be exercised. We have already discussed using a fitball in daily work situations. Another good habit is to bend your knees and squat instead of bending from the waist. Always sit with your back straight. Try and use the squatting position as much as possible for daily activities. All these activities strengthen muscles and ligaments relevant to maintaining continence.

几乎所有的症状都消失了,在 4 年后的最后一次随访时也是如此。

对后部韧带症状非手术治疗的点评

来就诊的许多患者通过像 B 小姐采用的治疗方法,尤其是用健身球代替椅子,使盆腔疼痛、尿急、排尿异常和夜尿等症状得到了很大改善。这种方法非常省时,对绝经前的中青年女性尤其有效。

对盆底训练在当今失禁治疗中地位的点评

盆底肌和其他肌肉群一样,是身体的一部分,也需要接受训练。我们已经讨论过在日常工作中使用健身球训练,另一个好习惯是弯曲膝盖后下蹲,而不是弯腰。坐时始终保持背部挺直。日常活动中尽量采用下蹲动作。上述所有动作都能增强与控尿相关的肌肉和韧带的功能。

(上海交通大学医学院附属第六人民医院妇产科,邱雨 译,吴氢凯 校)

CHAPTER 7 Constipation and Fecal Incontinence Haemorrhoids and Anal Fissures

SPECIAL CONTRIBUTION by Dr Darren Gold MSc MB ChB FRCS (Gen) FRCS (Eng) FRACS
Coloproctologist, Colorectal Surgeon and Pelvic Reconstructive Surgeon

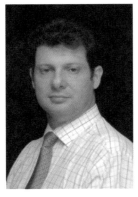

Dr Gold is a Senior Lecturer in Surgery at St Vincent's Clinical School, UNSW, and has a private practice at 193 Macquarie St Sydney where he works as a Colorectal Surgeon and also, in Female Pelvic Floor reconstruction with Professor Petros. Dr Gold is the Secretary for the International Society of Pelviperineology, and was one of the founder members of the South of England Pelvic Floor Group. He is fully trained in the TFS and Integral Theory System of diagnosis and surgery. Dr Gold has given numerous international lectures in his subspecialist surgical field, constipation, faecal incontinence, haemorrhoids, anal pain, anal fissure, pilonidal sinus, anal fistula, proctology and inflammatory bowel disease (Crohn's disease and Ulcerative Colitis).

Dr. Gold qualified from London University in 1989. He spent 11years undertaking his surgical training, including at the iconic StMark's Hospital in London. In 2000, he was appointed as a consultant colorectal surgeon at Basingstoke Hospital in Hampshire, an internationally recognised unit for the management of cancer of the colon and rectum. Subsequently he emigrated to Sydney with his Australian wife.

第七章　便秘、粪失禁、痔疮和肛裂

特邀撰稿人：Darren Gold 医生，理学硕士，医学学士，外科学学士，皇家外科医学院荣誉院士（德国），皇家外科医学院荣誉院士（英国），澳大利亚皇家外科医学院荣誉院士，结直肠病专家，结直肠外科和盆腔重建外科医生。

Gold 医生是新南威尔士大学（University of New South Wales, UNSW）、圣文森特临床医学院（St Vincent's Clinical School）的外科学高级讲师，并在悉尼麦格理街 193 号（193 Macquarie St Sydney）私人执业。在那里，他是一名结直肠外科医生，同时与 Petros 教授一起从事女性盆底重建工作。Gold 医生是国际盆底会阴学协会（the International Society of Pelviperine-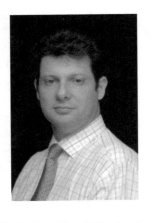
ology）的学术秘书，也是南英格兰盆底学组（South of England Pelvic Floor Group）的创始人之一。他完整地接受了 TFS 悬吊系统和应用"整体理论系统"诊断和手术的培训。Gold 医生在他的亚专科手术领域做过许多国际演讲，包括便秘、粪失禁、痔疮、肛门疼痛、肛裂、藏毛窦（pilonidal sinus。译者注：藏毛窦是在骶尾部臀间裂软组织内的一种慢性窦道或囊肿，内藏毛发是其特征）、肛瘘、直肠病和炎症性肠病（克罗恩病和溃疡性结肠炎）。

Gold 医生于 1989 年从伦敦大学毕业。他花了 11 年时间接受外科训练，包括在伦敦著名的圣马克医院（St Mark's Hospital）工作。2000 年，他被任命为汉普郡贝辛斯托克医院（Basingstoke Hospital in Hampshire）的结直肠外科顾问，这是一个国际闻名的结肠癌和直肠癌诊治中心。随后，他随澳大利亚籍妻子移居悉尼。

Introduction

A holistic perspective

We have found that the conditions detailed below are often caused by loose back ligaments and perineal body. They are often associated with bladder problems and chronic pain, but with a different emphasis. For example, chronic severe pain in the tailbone is far more commonly associated with problems such as haemorrhoidsand anal fissures, than with bladder problems. As the causes of these conditions are many and varied, it is important to find exactly what is causing the problem before treatment can commence.

Constipation is when the stools are hard, difficult to pass and not regular, often several days apart. The causes of constipation can vary from congenital absence in the nerve supply to the bowel wall, to a slow passage through the bowel of food. Many patients with constipation from these causes will frequently have symptoms either in childhood or teenage years and the situation will be well established by middle age.

Faecal incontinence is the inability to control the stools with loss of liquid or solid into the underwear. Many women have perfectly normal bowel function until the menopause or a hysterectomy, at which point symptoms of constipation and faecal incontinence, or sometimes both will suddenly occur. The causes of such constipation are different to those which occur in childhood, as they would have been obvious years earlier.

The sudden appearance of such symptoms is often embarrassing. If the incontinence is severe, many women will never seek advice from a Doctor nor discuss it with their friends, a self-imposed "Conspiracy of Silence". Nonetheless symptoms such as these are exceptionally common. Many women find that they are aware of the need to pass a stool but are unable to do so. This gives an uncomfortable feeling of fullness and a feeling that the bowel is never successfully emptied properly. These symptoms are known

导言

一种整体的视角

我们发现,以下所描述的病情经常是由后部韧带和会阴体松弛造成的,并常常和膀胱问题及慢性盆腔疼痛相关,但是相关的程度有所不同。例如,骶尾骨慢性剧烈的疼痛更多与痔疮出血和肛裂有关,与膀胱问题相关性较小。由于这些病情的原因多种多样,在治疗之前找到准确的病因非常重要。

便秘是指粪便过硬、难于排出、排便不规律,经常几天才排便一次。便秘的原因各有不同,可能是直肠壁神经的先天性缺陷,也可能是因为食物通过肠道缓慢。这些原因会导致许多人在儿童期或青少年期就经常出现便秘,并持续至中年。

粪失禁是指无法控制稀便或者成形粪便排在内裤上。许多女性原本排便功能完好,但到围绝经期或者子宫切除之后,出现便秘、粪失禁或者有时两者同时出现。这类便秘和童年期便秘的原因不同,因为后者在很多年前就已有明显的便秘症状。

突然出现这些症状会令人非常尴尬。如果失禁严重,许多女性既不寻求医生的建议,也不和朋友讨论——一种强加于自己的"缄默的密约"。尽管如此,这些症状还是很常见的。不少女性能感觉到便意,但是排不出粪便。这种情况下,患者会因为粪便胀满而不适,有种肠道永远不能正常排空的感觉。这些症状就是"排便障碍综合征(obstructed defecation syndrome,ODS)"。许多患者将其描述为一种阻碍粪便顺利排出的阻塞感。

那么,为什么许多女性会在围绝经期或者子宫切除之后突

as "obstructed defecation syndrome" as many women will describe it as a feeling of blockage that prevents the stool from passing successfully.

So why do so many women suddenly suffer from constipation and faecal incontinence around the menopause or following a hysterectomy? The reason for this is very similar to why women develop bladder problems after the menopause or hysterectomy, the ligaments become weak.

The same ligaments that support the vagina and bladder also support the bowel and anus. The back ligaments are the main supports of the bowel as regards emptying it and closing it.

Frequently during childbirth, the back ligaments are stretched and damaged. The main support of the ligaments is collagen. Collagen acts like the steel rods in cement. The hormones oestrogen and testosterone keep the collagen strong. At the menopause, the ovaries suddenly decrease production of oestrogen. The ligaments, deprived of oestrogen weaken and can no longer support the organs or the muscles, so prolapse of the bowel wall may appear. These same ligaments have to be cut to remove the uterus during a hysterectomy, which is why the symptoms may appear so suddenly.

If the back ligaments are weak, the patient has to strain hard to empty. This further weakens the vagina so it can no longer support the bowel. The bowel balloons into the vagina as a lump called a rectocele. The stool may enter the lump instead of passing through. This further increases the feeling of fullness.

The anus is also important for the bowel to empty. It must open for the stool to pass, but it must also be held in a fixed position as the stool is passing through it.

It is the perineal body, the thick lump of tissue between the anus and the vagina, which holds the anus in position. The perineal body is crucial for passing stools in a normal way. Frequently at childbirth the head overstretches the perineal body, so it becomes loose, so it moves during evacuation. This prevents the stool from passing easily. As it, too, contains large amounts of collagen, it will also weaken at the menopause.

然出现便秘和粪失禁呢？这和同样情况下出现膀胱问题的原因非常相似，即后部韧带松弛。

支持阴道和膀胱的韧带与支持直肠肛门的韧带是相似的。后部韧带是支持直肠的主要韧带，主要负责开放和闭合直肠。

分娩时，后部韧带经常被过度牵拉和损伤。韧带中主要的支持结构是胶原蛋白，胶原蛋白的作用类似于水泥中的钢筋。雌激素和雄激素使胶原蛋白保持张力。在围绝经期，卵巢产生的雌激素突然降低，韧带由于缺乏雌激素变得薄弱，不再能支持盆腔器官和肌肉，于是出现直肠壁脱垂。子宫切除术中，在切除子宫时这些韧带被一并切断，这也是以上症状会突然出现的原因。

假如后部韧带薄弱了，患者就得用力屏气才能排便，这样会使阴道变得更薄弱，进一步减弱了对肠道的支持作用。肠道就会像块物一样突入阴道，这被称为直肠膨出。粪便可能进入疝囊而无法排出，更加重了肠道胀满感。

肛门在排便过程中也是至关重要的，它不仅必须保持开放，还必须保持在一个固定的位置。

会阴体是位于肛门和阴道之间的一块厚厚的组织，负责固定肛门的位置。会阴体对于正常的排便至关重要。分娩时，胎头的娩出常常过度伸展会阴体，使其变得松弛，导致在排便时会阴体位置发生变动，因此无法顺利排便。会阴体也含有大量胶原蛋白，所以在围绝经期同样会变得薄弱。

会阴体的作用类似于肌肉的锚定点，在排便后闭合肛门，避免粪便漏出。会阴体松弛会导致轻微的粪漏。很多女性在排便后不久会发现内裤上有一点脏，甚至有粪便。这就解释了为何那么多围绝经期女性会抱怨同时存在便秘和粪失禁症状，而许多医生认为这种情况是矛盾的。这些症状并存的原因其实很简

The perineal body acts as an anchor point for the muscles that close the anus after the bowel empties, so that it does not leak after emptying. A loose perineal body can cause some minor leakage of the bowel and many women find that there is some staining in their underwear or even loss of faeces shortly after they empty their bowels. This explains why many menopausal women can complain of simultaneous constipation and faecal incontinence which many medical practitioners find contradictory. The ability of these symptoms to coincide is explained simply by the fact that the back ligaments are the key support for the muscles which open and close the bowel.

Because the woman strains excessively to pass stools, the pressure blocks the veins and makes them swell up to cause haemorrhoids and even cause the lining of the bowel tissue to come out through the anus. As a result of the excessive movement of the anus during a bowel motion due to looseness of the perineal body, the anal tissues stretch unnaturally. The stretching and stress causing the delicate lining to tear is what causes an anal fissure.

Many women who had never previously experienced any problems at all from haemorrhoids or anal fissures suddenly find the symptoms appear at the same time as the constipation and incontinence, again a result of loose back ligaments and perineal body.

We have found that repair of the back ligaments and perineal body restores much needed support to the rectum, anus, and vagina. This support will frequently improve both the constipation and the incontinence and indeed, sexual intercourse. The haemorrhoids and anal fissures will also frequently disappear and the bowel can empty normally once more.

Haemorrhoids are usually caused by a combination of factors: straining, hard stools, poor diet. The most common cause in men is excessive straining at stool. In women, the most important cause is childbirth. Childbirth loosens the ligaments which hold up the bowel from the top and the perineal body which supports it from below. The veins in the lower bowel do not have any valves, so any looseness in the tissues may cause a blockage in the veins and this may distend into the bowel to cause discomfort and bleeding. The bleeding is bright red and associated with the bowel motion. Of course constipation and straining will greatly worsen this situation.

单，即后部韧带是支持肌肉的关键结构，而这些肌肉恰恰控制着直肠的开闭。

由于女性在排便时过度屏气，腹压增加，静脉回流受阻，静脉隆起形成痔疮，甚至造成直肠黏膜外翻。松弛的会阴体导致排便时肛门的过度移动，肛门组织非自然地伸展。伸展和腹压引起脆弱的黏膜发生撕裂，导致肛裂。

那些之前从未经历过痔疮和肛裂的女性，会突然发现这些症状和便秘、失禁同时出现，这同样是后部韧带和会阴体松弛的结果。

我们发现，修复后部韧带和会阴体能重建对直肠、肛门和阴道的必要支撑，这些支撑力通常能改善便秘、失禁甚至提高性生活质量。痔疮和肛裂往往随之消失，排便恢复正常。

痔疮通常是由于以下几个原因引起：屏气、粪便干结、不合理饮食。男性痔疮的主要原因是排便时过度屏气。对于女性而言，主要原因是阴道分娩。阴道分娩使得从上方牵引肠道的韧带和从下方承托肠道的会阴体都松弛了。肠道下段的静脉没有静脉瓣，所以任何组织的松弛都可能导致静脉淤滞，进而膨胀入肠道，引起不适和出血。这样的出血是鲜红色的，并和排便有关。当然，便秘和屏气将极大地加重这种病情。

Warning- not all bleeding is caused by haemorrhoids

The symptoms listed below may be caused by more serious conditions, including cancer:
* The blood is dark
* Bleeding occurs independent of opening the bowel
* Blood seen on or in the stool
* Change in bowel habit
* Weight loss
* Loss of appetite
* Abdominal pain or distension

Treatment for haemorrhoids

Many patients will respond to conservative measures. The most important is avoidance of straining and allowing the stool to come out normally. This means if on sitting on the toilet the bowel does not empty, do not strain. Get up and come back later. Adding bulk to the diet such as wheat bran, fruit and vegetables or even natural aperients. Local treatments such as astringents, cortisone etc. should be given under doctor's orders. If the condition persists, it may require specialized treatment, usually by a coloproctologist.

Anal fissures

An anal fissure is a split in the lining of the anal tube. Constipation is an important cause. The main symptom is pain on opening the bowel associated with a small stain of bright blood. This pain is often severe. The pain usually lasts a week or two, but with ointments and stool softeners, the fissure usually heals within two weeks. If the condition persists, it may require specialized treatment, usually by a coloproctologist.

注意：不是所有的出血都是由痔疮引起的

以下列出的症状可能由更严重的病因所致，包括恶性肿瘤：
- 暗红色出血
- 出血和排便没有关联
- 血迹在粪便表面或内部
- 排便习惯改变
- 消瘦
- 食欲缺乏
- 腹痛或腹胀

痔疮的治疗

许多患者保守治疗有效，其最重要的措施是避免屏气，尽量自然排便。这意味着当您坐上马桶感觉大便未排净时，不要用力屏气。应该站起来，过一会儿再回来尝试。可以在饮食中增加如麦麸、水果和蔬菜的食用量，甚至服用天然的轻泻剂。收敛剂、类固醇等局部治疗的药物，应在医生的指导下使用。如果症状不见好转，则需接受专科治疗，通常由结直肠科医生治疗。

肛裂

肛裂是指肛管内的黏膜发生撕裂，主要的起因是便秘。主要的症状是排便时疼痛，伴有少量鲜血。这种疼痛往往是剧烈的，通常持续1～2周。使用软膏和粪便软化剂后，肛裂往往能在2周内自愈。如果症状不见好转，则需接受专科治疗，通常由结直肠科医生治疗。

Chronic pain and other symptoms associated with these

We have found that these conditions are usually associated with pain of varying severity in the tail bone, lower abdomen or even the entrance to the vagina. On questioning, these patients may have other bowel problems and bladder symptoms such as nocturia, urgency, frequency or stress incontinence.

INDIVIDUAL STORIES
From our Macquarie St Clinic
Severe painful anal fissure from chronic constipation

Mrs C stated *"I have suffered from Chronic Constipation for many years which resulted in a fissure (internal and external) causing severe anal pain and bladder weakness. Despite several consultations with General Practitioners and specialists, the problem had not been satisfactorily resolved"*
Mrs C came to our clinic via the Internet. She continues
"After my first consultation, an admission was arranged to the hospital for day surgery consisting of a Botox injection to paralyse the area to allow healing. It was explained to me that whereas this would ease the pain for some months, it did not address the underlying cause of the problem."
Because Mrs C had other pelvic symptoms, I arranged a joint consultation with my colleague Professor Peter Petros, a gynaecologist who, like me, specializes in pelvic floor reconstruction. We have found joint consultations to be immensely useful, as patients with bowel problems such as chronic constipation, faecal incontinence, haemorrhoids and fissures, almost without exception, have other pelvic floor problems such as pain, bladder symptoms, or vaginal prolapse.
We found that total prolapse (bladder, vagina and bowel). We recommended pelvic repair surgery to repair all the ligaments,

慢性疼痛和其他相关的症状

我们发现,这些病情通常和不同程度的尾骨疼痛、下腹痛甚至阴道口疼痛有关。问题是,这些患者可能同时伴有其他的排便、排尿问题,如夜尿、尿频、急迫性或者压力性尿失禁。

个案故事
来自我们的麦格理街诊所(Macquarie St Clinic)
由慢性便秘引起的严重肛裂疼痛

C 太太说:"多年来,我饱受慢性便秘之苦,并引起内、外肛裂,继而出现严重的肛门疼痛和膀胱无力。尽管我曾经就诊于多位全科医生和专科医生,但病痛的问题一直都未得到圆满解决。"

C 太太通过互联网找到了我们诊所,她说:

"在初次就诊后,我被安排住院进行一次日间手术,在疼痛部位注射肉毒杆菌素使局部神经麻痹,以利痊愈。他们向我解释,虽然术后几个月可以缓解疼痛,但并没有解决根本的病因。

由于 C 太太还有其他的盆腔症状,我安排了一次和我的同事 Peter Petros 教授的联合会诊。Peter Petros 教授是一位妇科专家,像我一样专注于盆底重建领域的工作。我们发现联合会诊很有意义,因为这些患有慢性便秘、粪失禁、痔疮和肛裂等排便问题的患者,几乎无一例外地伴随其他的盆腔问题,如疼痛、膀胱症状或者阴道脱垂。

我们发现她患有全盆底器官脱垂(膀胱、阴道和直肠),因此建议通过盆底手术修复所有的韧带,包括前部、中部、后部韧带

front, middle and back and also, perineal body. The procedure was jointly carried out by both surgeons.

She continues *"I remained in hospital for 2 days and was then discharged. The procedure has proved to be fully successful. I am pain free, my bladder and bowels now work perfectly and I now have my normal life back. I wish to express my sincere thanks to my doctors for an amazing result. "*

Severe bowel and bladder incontinence

Mrs JR stated *" Mine is a personal and generally a very private story within the community, however my life has been changed so dramatically and positively for the better since treatment, I believe the history should be shared.*

I am a female of 72 years. For most of my adult life, I have worked as a Pharmacist, so I have some knowledge of incontinence problems. For at least the last 10 years, I have been incontinent, affecting both my bladder and to some extent bowels.

Despite having a wide circle of close female friends I was unwilling because of embarrassment to share the extent of my ongoing misery.

I did seek medical treatment in 2004 from a well-known clinic but the only option offered was pelvic floor exercises used to strengthen the pelvic floor muscles. Despite my best efforts little relief was gained. In 2008, my bowel prolapsed ("turned inside out"). I had an operation in 2009 with another surgeon which helped the bowel prolapse, but it did nothing for my bowel and bladder incontinence which gradually got worse. I had problems emptying my bladder and suffered from bladder infections.

Anyone who is unfortunate enough to suffer these problems knows of the inconvenience of needing to be aware of the location of public toilets when shopping, or visiting theatres or any function. Pads have to be worn continually, need to be disposed of

以及会阴体。手术由我和 Peter Petros 医生共同完成。

她继续说："*我在医院住了两天就出院了。结果证明手术很成功，现在疼痛消失了，膀胱和肠道功能完好，我已经回归正常的生活。我希望以此向我的医生们表达最真挚的谢意，感谢他们给了我令人惊喜的疗效。*"

严重的肠道和膀胱失禁

JR 太太说："*就社会大众的眼光来看，我的经历总体算是一个非常隐私的故事。自从接受治疗后，我的生活发生了如此戏剧性且积极的改善，所以我相信，应该与大家分享这段经历。*"

我是一名 72 岁的女性。在成年后的大部分时间里是一名药剂师，所以对大小便失禁有所了解。在过去至少 10 年里，我一直有大小便失禁症状，影响膀胱且在某种程度上影响肠道。

尽管有很多闺蜜，我还是会因为尴尬而不愿意向她们倾诉自己正在遭遇的痛苦。

我曾在 2004 年到一家著名的诊所求医，但唯一的选择是只能通过盆底训练来加强盆底肌肉。尽管我已竭尽全力，但仍收效甚微。2008 年，我得了肠脱垂（内面翻到了外面）。2009 年我接受过一次手术，由另一名外科医生帮我治疗脱垂，但粪、尿失禁并没有改善，病情每况愈下。不仅膀胱很难排空，还反复感染。

任何正在遭遇此等不幸的人都相当清楚生活的不便，在购物场所、剧院或从事任何社交活动时，都必须知道公厕的位置。护垫要一直戴着，小心翼翼地处理掉，希望不要被人察觉到异

discreetly, and one is very cognisant of unwanted odour and heaven forbid, "accidents", not only urine, but bowel soiling, often in the most inconvenient places.

Last year a friend offered the advice that new treatment was available in Australia, and that she had been cured. When my husband had to have a radical prostatectomy and he too became incontinent, I became more aware of the huge impact that this problem causes to numerous other lives. I realised it was time to investigate again."

Mrs R saw us in our Macquarie St Clinic at a joint consultation. It was evident that she had loose ligaments in the front and back and also, her perineal body was loose. Her front and back ligaments and perineal body were repaired with the TFS system which repairs only the damaged ligaments. Six months later she stated,

"The result has been remarkable. There is now no leakage from the bladder or bowel and I am emptying my bladder normally. There have been no further bladder infections."

Descending Perineum Syndrome

This condition occurs when the tissue joining the two perineal bodies is destroyed, usually at childbirth. What happens is that the head descends downwards like a bulldozer and it pushes the perineal bodies to the side, so the rectum now protrudes upwards as a lump called a rectocele. The rectal tissue can also fold inwards to block descent of the feces. This causes the patient to feel that there is an obstruction inside.

The main symptoms are inability to empty the bowel because of obstruction, constipation and fecal incontinence, both a result of looseness in the back ligaments and/or perineal body. When the patient strains, the anus can be seen to descend several centimeters down. At present, this condition is considered to be incurable. This is incorrect. We use the TFS technique, a minimally invasive method which links the separated perineal bodies with a tape. When the tape

味。常常在最不方便的场合,尿液甚至粪便会意外地漏出来。

去年,一位朋友向我提议,澳大利亚有新的治疗方法,她通过治疗已经痊愈了。我的丈夫在做了根治性前列腺切除术后也出现了失禁,这越发让我意识到它对无数人的生活造成了巨大的影响。我明白是时候再去彻底检查一次了。

R 太太在麦格理街诊所(Macquarie St Clinic)接受了联合会诊。很明显,她的前部韧带和后部韧带以及会阴体都松弛了。我们仅使用了 TFS 系统修复受损的前部、后部韧带和会阴体。6 个月后,她说:

"疗效非常显著。现在我不再漏尿、漏粪了,排尿正常,膀胱感染再也没有发生过。"

会阴下降综合征

这种情况发生在连接左右两侧会阴体的组织被破坏时,通常由阴道分娩造成。分娩时胎头下降,像推土机一样将会阴体向两边推开,导致直肠向上突起,形成直肠膨出。直肠组织向内折叠,阻止粪便排出,患者也会感觉到阻塞感。

梗阻、便秘和粪失禁引起的主要症状是粪便无法排空,这是由后部韧带和(或)会阴体松弛造成的。患者屏气时,肛门会下降数厘米。目前,这种情况往往被认为是无法治愈的,但事实并非如此。我们应用 TFS 这种微创技术将分离的会阴体用吊带连接起来。调整吊带,把两侧分离的会阴体上提并连接在一起。这样,肠道就被推向后方,并保持位置。患者的症状将显著改善,可以正常排便而无须借助手的按压。

is adjusted, it lifts the separated perineal bodies upwards and joins them together. This action pushes the bowel backwards and keeps it there. The patients experience a remarkable disappearance of their symptoms. The bowel can now empty properly, without the need for a patient to put her hand down to assist the emptying.

We received this letter from an American patient, a specialist doctor who had this condition. She communicated with us and we referred her to a Urology colleague in Minnesota USA.

I had episiotomy done during my first delivery that completely destroyed my perineum. I developed descending perineum syndrome, fecal incontinence and obstructed defecation. I sought help in many major american universities-UMDNJ, NYU, Mayo Clinic, Cleveland Clinic, University of Iowa, University of Oklahoma and I have been in correspondence with many more. I had an excruciatingly painful perineorrhaphy that fell apart after three months and another perineorrhaphy and posterior colporrhaphy a year later that fell apart after four months and left me with even less support. After all these repairs the defecography showed 7cm rectal descent and the notes from my ob-gyn state "the perineal body is very short, separated fascia". It came to a point I could hardly sit any more as I was sitting on my rectum. I was told by University of Iowa, where I had the last repair, and by everybody else that no further repair is possible. In desperation I wrote to Dr. Peter Petros who's innovative methods have caught my attention. He reviewed all my tests and questions, full of compassion and support, as I was so beaten up by the painful futile surgeries. He got me in touch with a surgeon in University of Minneapolis who works with his methods. He communicated with me during my recovery providing expert advice. Four months after his TFS sling repair the defecography showed no perineal/ rectal descent neither at rest or with Valsalva. The notes of my local ob-gyn state "the perienum looks normal, has good support".

It is not possible to express my gratitude to Dr. Petros who reached out to me from the other side of the planet to help.

我们接到一位美国患者的来信,她是一位患有此病的专科医生。沟通之后,我们将她介绍给了美国明尼苏达州的泌尿科同行。

　　我在第一次分娩时做了会阴侧切,但会阴体还是被完全破坏了,并最后进展为会阴下降综合征,出现了粪失禁和排便障碍。在美国,我已在许多著名的大学和医院求医,包括新泽西医科与牙科大学(UMDNJ)、纽约大学(NYU)、梅奥诊所(Mayo Clinic)、克利夫兰诊所(Cleveland Clinic)、爱荷华州大学(University of Iowa)、俄克拉荷马大学(University of Oklahoma)等。我曾经接受了一次疼痛难忍的会阴修补术,可术后3个月就裂开了。一年后又进行了一次会阴修补和阴道后壁修补手术,结果4个月后它再次开裂,支撑的组织更加薄弱。经历所有这些修复术后,排粪造影显示我的直肠下降了7厘米,妇产科检查显示:"会阴体过短,筋膜分离"。那段时间我到了几乎不能坐下去的地步,因为我就坐在自己的直肠上。我最后一次修复手术是在爱荷华大学(University of Iowa),所有人都告诉我,不可能再修复了。绝望中,Peter Petros医生的创新方法引起了我的注意。我向他写信,他一一询问了我所有的检查结果和病情,言语间充满着同情和支持,毕竟我被痛苦而徒劳的手术折磨着。他让我联系了明尼阿波利斯大学(University of Minneapolis)的一位外科医生,那位医生也采用他的方法治疗。康复期间,他也与我保持沟通,提供专业的意见。在TFS修复术后4个月,排粪造影显示,静息或向下屏气动作时,会阴和直肠都没有下降,妇科检查显示:"会阴体外观正常,支持力良好"。

　　Peter Petros医生从地球的另一边向我伸出援手,我对他的感激之情无法言喻。多亏了他毕生的努力,使像我这样因分

*Thanks to his lifelong efforts women like me with severe pelvic
floor damage sustained during childbirth will have a chance to feel
like human beings again.*

(Dr) B. K. , MD

Mrs S was an extraordinary patient. She had been given up as
impossible to cure by every expert in the pelvic floor field in
Sydney.
When we examined her, all the ligaments on the right hand side
had been ruptured, to the point where the organs were skewed to
the right side.

*My story began when I was 5 years old when I got caught up in a
swimming pool cleaner. It literally sucked out my insides so they
were hanging out of my vagina. I was admitted as an emergency
to the hospital and almost died. I was saved by the skill of the
surgeons, and escaped with the loss of some of my bowel.*

*Fast forward to my 30s. I was in a desperate situation. Neither
my bowel nor my bladder was working properly. I was wet with
urine, could not hang on, had to get up several times a night. My
bowel was constipated. I leaked faeces. I had terrible pain in my
pelvis. I could not have sexual intercourse.*

*Until meeting you, I was a broken mess, trying to hide just how
desperately worried I was about my future and scared to even hope
that I could be fixed. My husband was convinced I could if we just
found the right doctor smart enough to put it all together. After
others had scratched their heads and pronounced me a mystery (a
phrase a patient never wants to hear unless someone's prepared to
stick around and solve it) when x-ray, ultrasounds, CT Scans,
MRIs, colonoscopies, endoscopie, hospitalization for kidney
failure after too many antibiotics, every blood test under the sun,*

娩受到严重盆底损伤的妇女,能够获得重生。

B. K 医生

S 太太是一位特别的患者。悉尼盆底领域的每一位专家都认为她是不可能治愈的。

检查时,我们发现她右侧所有的韧带都离断了,以至于所有的器官都歪向了右侧。

我的故事开始于 5 岁的时候,当时我被一个泳池内的清洁器吸住,它几乎把我的内脏全部从阴道吸出。我当时被紧急送往医院,差一点失去生命。外科医生用精湛的技术把我救了回来,虽然逃离了死神,但我还是被切除了部分肠管。

快到 30 岁时。我的处境令人绝望,肠道和膀胱都不能正常工作了。我无法憋尿,总是会尿湿,夜里不得不多次起床。我有便秘,同时却会发生粪便漏出,盆腔疼痛严重,还无法进行性生活。

在遇见您之前,我的人生已经破碎不堪,我只能极力掩饰对自己的未来是多么的绝望,甚至已经害怕到不敢想象自己还有被治愈的希望。我丈夫却相信,如果我们能找到一位合适的、技术精湛的医生,我的人生可以重回正轨。医生们挠着头说我是个谜(除非有医生愿意留下来解决这个问题,否则没有患者想听到这个词)。当我经历了 X 线、超声、CT 扫描、磁共振成像、结肠镜、胃镜检查,因为过度使用抗生素致肾衰竭而住院,不断地抽血化验,理疗师、针灸师、营养师都一筹莫展,我的斗志理所当然地被消磨殆尽。在一位知名专家吹捧的粪便微生物移植

physio, acupuncture and dieticians had all drawn blanks, understandably my morale was waning. After a Fecal Microbiotia Transplant touted by a pop-star specialist as my cure-all did nothing (except finish off my savings), I finally learned to stop getting my hopes up and not buy into flashy promises.

So when I finally had my consultation, the manner of the doctors was so spot on, it was a relief in itself. The "no promises, no predictions" tact immediately gave me a feeling of trust, which was furthered by the cautious and methodical investigation which was mapped out, dotting all the is and crossing all the ts to get to the bottom of the mystery.

This conscientious approach took an immediate psychological strain off. For the first time, I felt confident that a medical professional really had my best interests at heart and wasn't just pushing their own agenda. I was deeply impressed by the combined team approach involving multiple doctors which again furthered my trust and respect knowing that multiple brains were taking part in solving the puzzle.

So by the time it had been worked out that surgery was my best option, I felt completely confident in you all, no matter what the outcome.

And then, blow me down if you all didn't all go and fix me. I am speechless. Every single symptom has been cured. I am speechless!

It feels nothing short of miraculous and I keep pinching myself to see that I'm not dreaming. However, by the 4th week mark, I had to say that the changes were absolutely undeniable. I'm just amazed and so excited about what the future holds now that I have one again.

术对我也无济于事(除了把我的积蓄花光)之后,我终于学会了不再抱有奢望,不再去相信那些华而不实的承诺。

所以,当我终于接受会诊时,医生们的态度是如此的到位,这本身就是一种解脱。"没有承诺,没有预期"的得体沟通立刻给了我一种信任的感觉,而这种信任又被精心安排好的、谨慎而有条理的检查所推动,一丝不苟地寻找到谜团背后的真相。

这种认真的态度立即消除了我心理上的压力。我第一次感到自信的是,一位医学专家真的把我的最大利益放在心上,而不仅仅自行其事地推动他们自己的进程。多名医生参与的团队合作方式再次加深了我对他们的信任和尊重,这给我留下了深刻的印象,因为我知道,多个大脑正在共同参与解决这个难题。

所以经过探讨,手术成为最佳选择方案时,无论结果如何,我都对你们充满信任。

当时,如果你们不给我治疗,我将无所适从。我激动得说不出话,现在每一个症状都被治愈了,我简直说不出话来!

这简直就是个奇迹,我不断地掐自己来确定这不是在做梦。而且,在术后第四周,我不得不说这种改变是毋庸置疑的。我惊讶并兴奋地对未来充满期待,那是我再次拥有的未来。

谢谢!这两个字不足以表达我的感谢之情。感谢你们鼓起勇气,在传统医学现状之外的探索工作,并且站在了令人惊叹

Thank you. These two words just don't begin to cover it. Thank you for your guts to explore work outside of the old-fashioned medical status quo and be at the forefront of something amazing. Thank you for your generosity which enabled my surgery.

You are an extraordinary lot. I am so humbled by this whole process. Whatever I can do to help further the cause you be sure to to let me know. Use my real name in the study. I have proudly had my bottom tied in a bow and my innards restrung.
Forever grateful.

We used the TFS system to precisely create artificial ligaments to replace those which had been torn. Though we state in the last chapter that it is possible to use older substitute operations, none of these older surgical methods would have been even remotely applicable here. Because she was young and her muscles undamaged, once we repaired the ligaments, the muscles could now work properly: all her symptoms were cured.

的技术前沿。

感谢你们的慷慨，促成了我的手术。

你们是非凡的一群人，整个过程让我受宠若惊。无论我能做些什么来帮助这个事业的发展，请一定告诉我。请在研究中使用我的真名。非常自豪的是，我的盆底重新收紧，内脏再也不会掉出来了。

永远感激！

我们应用组织固定系统（TFS）精准地重建人工韧带以替换那些被撕脱的韧带。虽然我们在最后一章中指出，应用传统的替代手术也是可取的，但在这个病例中，这些老的手术方法必将收效甚微。因为她还年轻，肌肉没有损伤，所以一旦我们修复了韧带，肌肉就可以正常工作了：她的所有症状都被治愈了。

（上海交通大学医学院附属第六人民医院妇产科，陈立奇 译，张睿 校）

CHAPTER 8   Nutrition and General Care for Incontinence

Diet is very helpful for bowel problems, but it is not so helpful with bladder problems. However, depending on the individual, avoiding certain foods may assist the worsening of bladder symptoms.

Do not reduce water intake—manage it The body needs about 8 glasses of water per day to function properly. It is required for digestion, adequate blood circulation, excretion and absorption of water soluble vitamins. Water is also required to make saliva, fluid for the joints and for the regulation of body temperature. Yet most women with bladder control problems reduce the amount of liquids they drink so that they will control their bladder in a better way. This is not unexpected, as those women who have stress incontinence lose more urine with a larger bladder volume. It is the same with the problem of urge incontinence. The emptying reflex is triggered at a smaller bladder volume than in normal women. Whereas reducing fluid intake can be effective, indeed, advisable, as a short term solution in a sensitive social situation, it is not advisable as a longer term strategy. Insufficient volume passing through the bladder can in some cases encourage the growth of bacteria, which can lead to infections. So the solution is to use common sense to manage the problem, ensuring that, by the end of the day, a full quota of fluids has been consumed.

Drinking a glass or two of water first thing on getting up in the morning will flush out the kidneys and the bladder. Then it is a matter of managing your fluid intake according to social needs, ensuring by the end of the day that you have drunk at least 2 litres of fluid.

Avoidance of certain foods and beverages Some foods or

第八章　营养和尿失禁的综合护理

　　饮食控制对改善肠道功能有很大的帮助，但对改善膀胱功能没有什么帮助。然而，避免摄入某些食物可以帮助一些人避免膀胱症状的恶化。

　　不要减少水的摄入——饮水管理　人体每天需要 8 杯水来维持正常工作。人体的消化吸收、充分的血液循环、排泄以及水溶性维生素的摄取都需要水。水也是生成唾液、关节润滑液、调节体温所必需的。但大部分有排尿问题的女性会减少水的摄入，以便更好地控制膀胱排尿。这并不令人惊讶，因为对于患有压力性尿失禁的女性来说，更大的膀胱容量意味着有更多的尿液溢出。急迫性尿失禁也是如此，与正常女性相比，更小的膀胱容量即可触发膀胱排空反射。尽管在敏感的社交情境下，减少液体摄入量作为短期解决方案确实有效，但是并不推荐作为长期策略。因为膀胱的排尿量不足有时会导致细菌滋生，从而引起感染。因此，解决方案是用科学的认识来管理这个问题，保证在一天结束时摄入足量的液体。早晨起床时先喝一两杯水冲洗肾脏和膀胱。然后根据社交需要来管理液体摄入，确保在一天结束时摄入至少 2 L 的液体。

　　避免某些食物和饮料　某些食物或饮料会刺激膀胱。这种情况的个体差异比较大，我们目前也不知道它是如何影响膀胱功能的。但对每位女性来说，有件事情非常重要，那就是观察哪些食物或饮料可能对膀胱功能造成负面影响，并避免摄入这些食物。茶、酒、咖啡等饮品可能导致多尿，使膀胱充盈更快，也可

beverages may cause irritation of the bladder. It is an individual thing, and how they affect the bladder is not always understood. It is a matter for each woman to observe what makes the bladder worse and eliminating or avoiding these items. Beverages such as tea, alcohol, coffee will cause excess production of urine and fill the bladder more rapidly, but are also likely to dehydrate the system, requiring a greater fluid intake. Acidic foods such as citrus and tomatoes, tea, coffee, corn syrup, artificial sweeteners such as aspartate, carbonated drinks such as diet cola, all may irritate the bladder. As we said, the irritants differ from person to person, so it is a matter of closely observing and avoiding any irritants. Some foods may cause diarrhoea or gas and so may worsen faecal incontinence if it is present. These include spicy foods, fatty and greasy foods, cured or smoked meat, carbonated beverages, and dairy products if a woman is lactose intolerant. Again, it is a matter of closely observing and avoiding.

Non-irritating thirst quenchers such as water itself, or fruit juices such as grape, apple and of course cranberry, are good to drink. These make the urine more acidic, which can prevent the spread of bacteria in the urinary tract. Bacteria may cause urinary tract infections, which themselves cause the urge to urinate. Cranberry juice is especially good, as it has been shown scientifically to actually help avoid bladder infections.

Diabetes Good control of sugar level is critical, as excretion of sugar into the bladder will facilitate multiplication of the bacteria.

Obesity is the enemy of continence and not only because the extra weight increases the pressure on the bladder but also because obese patients always have higher complications and less success with surgery. In general terms, it is helpful to have a balanced diet with adequate protein and lots of fresh vegetables, avoiding sugar, fats and carbohydrates in excess.

It is always good to consult a professional dietician to ensure that there are adequate micronutrients like Magnesium, Calcium, Vitamin B12, Vitamin C and Zinc in the diet.

能导致身体脱水,需要摄入更多液体。酸性食品(如柑橘、西红柿)、茶、咖啡、玉米糖浆、人造甜味剂(如天冬氨酸)、碳酸饮料(如无糖可乐)都可能刺激膀胱。正如我们所言,刺激性食物的影响因人而异,需注意观察,尽量避免。某些食物会引起腹泻和腹胀,并加重粪失禁。这些食物包括辛辣食品、脂肪和油腻的食物、腌肉或烟熏肉、碳酸饮料和乳制品(对乳糖不耐受的女性),也需注意观察,尽量避免。

没有刺激性的止渴饮料 例如,水或果汁(如葡萄汁、苹果汁),当然还有蔓越莓汁,这些都是很好的饮料。它们使尿液的酸性增强,可以防止细菌在尿路中播散。细菌可能引起尿路感染,而尿路感染本身会引起尿急症状。蔓越莓汁特别好,它已被科学证明有助于避免膀胱感染。

糖尿病 控制好血糖水平至关重要,尿液的含糖量增加会促进细菌繁殖。

肥胖 是尿控的大敌,不仅是因为超重增加膀胱的压力,还因为肥胖患者的手术并发症发生率更高,成功率更低。总而言之,摄入含有充足蛋白质和多种新鲜蔬菜的均衡饮食,避免过多的碳水化合物和脂肪,这些对患者都是有益的。

患者最好咨询专业的营养师,以确保饮食中含有足够的微量营养素,如镁、钙、维生素 B_{12}、维生素 C 和锌。

Fibre is essential for the intestinal tract. It helps make the stool soft and easier to control. Fibre is mainly found in fruits, vegetables, and whole-grain breads and cereals. Dieticians recommend 20 to 30 grams of fibre a day but it should not be added to the diet all at once, as too much fibre taken suddenly may cause uncomfortable bloating and gas. Eight glasses of water per day are required to process the fibre sufficiently to soften the stool.

Skin care is essential to avoid further problems if there is faecal incontinence. The skin around the anus must be kept as clean and dry as possible, so as to relieve discomfort and eliminate the odour associated with faecal incontinence.

It is recommended that the anal area be washed with water after each bowel movement. If available, use of a bidet after each bowel or incontinence episode is the ideal solution. Showering or soaking in a bath may also help.

Soap can dry and irritate the skin, so a non-irritating soap should be used if required. Rubbing with dry toilet paper can cause abraisons on the skin. Pre-moistened, alcohol-free towelettes or wipes may be a good alternative for cleaning the area.

It is important to dry thoroughly. It is best to allow the area to air-dry, but if time is of the essence, a good alternative is to gently pat the area dry with toilet paper or a clean washcloth.

A barrier cream helps keep irritated skin from having direct contact with faeces. It is important that the area be clean and dry before applying such creams. Non-medicated talcum powder applied to a well-dried skin is a good traditional method to help relieve anal discomfort.

Clothing needs to be loose and underwear should be cotton. Tight clothing can restrict airflow and so may worsen skin problems. Soiled underwear should be changed immediately

Absorbent pads and disposable underwear can also help manage the problem. It is important that pads or adult diapers have an absorbent layer on top, to help keep moisture away from the skin.

纤维素　对肠道功能至关重要。它有助于软化粪便和控制排便。纤维素主要存在于水果、蔬菜、全麦面包和谷类食品中。营养学家建议每天摄入 20～30 克纤维素，但不应一次性加入饮食中，因为一下子摄入过多的纤维素可能会引起腹胀和排气等不适。每天需要饮用 8 杯水来充分处理纤维素以软化粪便。

皮肤护理　对于粪失禁的患者，避免出现其他问题至关重要。肛周皮肤必须尽可能保持清洁和干燥，以减轻粪失禁引起的不适和异味。

建议每次排便后用清水冲洗肛门区域。如果条件允许，在每次排便或粪失禁发作后坐浴是理想的方法。淋浴或泡澡也可能有帮助。

肥皂　会引起皮肤干燥并刺激皮肤。因此如果必要的话，应使用无刺激性的肥皂。干燥的厕纸可能会擦伤皮肤。用无酒精的湿巾纸清洁该区域是很好的选择。

彻底干燥非常重要。最好让皮肤自然风干，如果时间不允许，可用卫生纸或干净毛巾轻柔地拍干皮肤也是不错的选择。

隔离霜　有助于防止敏感的皮肤与粪便直接接触。在涂抹隔离霜之前，保持肛周皮肤清洁、干燥非常重要。把非药用的滑石粉涂在干燥的皮肤上，是帮助缓解肛门不适的传统好方法。

衣着　要宽松，内衣应该是棉质的。紧身的衣物会影响空气的流通，使皮肤问题恶化。弄脏的内衣应及时更换。

吸水的护垫和一次性内裤　也对肛周皮肤护理有帮助。重要的是护垫或成人尿布的上层要有吸水垫，以隔开水分和皮肤。

（上海交通大学医学院附属第六人民医院妇产科，李洁　译，薛卓维　校）

CHAPTER 9   A Typical Visit to the clinic

In this next chapter, we present a patient's experience at the clinic in her own words.

I rang to make an appointment. After making the appointment, the secretary discussed with me how the clinic worked. She said she would send me an information pamphlet and a list of questions (questionnaire) concerning my bladder and bowel, which I was to complete at home in my own time and hand in on arrival for my first appointment. She explained that the answers to these questions would assist the doctor in diagnosing which parts of my pelvic floor had been damaged. I was to arrive "with a comfortably full bladder" and to bring a sample of urine for testing. She also sent me information pamphlets on the clinic.

Kvinno Centre
Specialising in women's health needs

WHAT IS THE PELVIC FLOOR?

The floor of your pelvis is made up of layers of muscle and other clastic tissucs. It strelches like a firm, supportive hammock from the pubic bone in the front to the tail bone at the back. Because you cannot see them, these muscles are often neglected-but they are some of the most important in a woman's

第九章　一次典型的就诊经历

这一章，我们用患者自己的语言来讲述她的就诊经历。

首先打电话预约。预约后，秘书告诉我诊所的工作流程。她说会寄给我一份有相关信息的小册子，以及一份关于膀胱和肠道功能的问卷调查表，我可以利用空余时间在家完成，在第一次按约就诊时上交。她解释说，这份问卷的答案将协助医生判断盆底的哪一部分发生损伤。在我到达诊所时，"膀胱应处于适度的充盈状态"，并带上尿液样本做检测。她还寄给我一些关于诊所的小册子。

Kvinno 中心
妇女健康专家

什么是盆底?

盆底(pelvic floor)由肌肉层和弹性组织构成。它就像一个稳固、有支撑力的吊床，从前面的耻骨一直伸展延伸到后面的尾骨。由于看不见它们，这些肌肉往往会被忽视——但它们是女性身体最重要的一部分，维持着膀胱、子宫和肠道的正

body. They hold the bladder, uterus and bowel in place. They also support the three passages leading out of the body-the urethra (through which you pass urine), the vagina and the anus (back passage).

Strings or loops of muscle fibres (sphincters) around these openings are like valves. For example, the urinary sphincter stops and starts the flow of urine.

WHAT HAPPENS IF MUSCLES AND LIGAMENTS ARE WEAK?

A number of things can cause your pelvic floor to weaken or sag:

- Pregnancy and childbirth
- Loss of elasticity in the vagina with age
- Being more that 10 kilograms overweight
- Changes to hormone levels at menopause
- Lack of general exercise

Comment

The Kvinno Centre (Kvinno means woman in Swedish) was the first clinic in the world to be based on the Integral System. Though it no longer exists as an entity in its original location, the Integral Diagnostic and Surgical System on which it was based is increasingly being applied, in various degrees, worldwide.

My first consultation

When I arrived for my first consultation, the secretary checked that I had completed my questionnaire and arranged for the nurse to test my urine. In the consulting room, the doctor read my referral letter and asked me what my problem was. He then asked

常位置,支持着通向体外的 3 个通道——尿道(排尿的通道)、阴道和肛门(后方的排粪通道)。

这些开口周围的肌纤维环(括约肌)就像阀门。例如,尿道括约肌负责尿流的开始和终止。

如果肌肉和韧带薄弱了会怎样?

许多情况会导致您的盆底支持结构变弱或下垂:
- 妊娠和分娩
- 随年龄增长,阴道失去弹性
- 体重超重大于 10 kg 以上
- 更年期激素水平的变化
- 缺乏日常运动

点评

Kvinno 中心(Kvinno 在瑞典语中是"女人"的意思)是世界上第一家应用"整体理论系统"的诊所。尽管原来的实体诊所早已不复存在,但是基于"整体理论系统"的整体诊断及手术系统正在全球范围内得到不同程度的应用。

我的第一次就诊

第一次就诊时,诊所的秘书核实了我已经完成的问卷调查表,并安排护士检测尿液。在诊室里,医生认真地阅读了我的转诊信,并询问了症状;以及一般病史,包括分娩史、手术史、过敏史、药物史和输血史;查看了我的问卷表并讨论了选项和答案。

about my general medical history, my childbirth, previous operations, allergies, medications, and transfusions. He then read the completed questionnaire and discussed the answers with me. The doctor explained that the purpose of the questions was to uncover abnormal symptoms which would also serve as a guide as to which part(s) of the vagina had been damaged. He showed me the diagram below and said,

"Don't worry about the detail, just look at the three columns. The ticks tell us where the problems are. You will see that there are three areas of potential damage, in the front, middle and back ligaments, with specific symptoms and prolapses related to each".

He then proceeded to tell me that a prolapse was a bulge in the vagina by the bladder, uterus or bowel. Pelvic floor laxities which can be repaired.

He referred again me to the diagnostic diagram.

For example, the first question in the questionnaire asks: *"Do you lose urine when you cough?"*

I had answered yes to this question. The doctor ticked the "stress incontinence" column and explained that I had a problem in the front ligament of the vagina.

Later in the questionnaire I answered that I felt that my bladder didn't empty adequately, that I had urgency, constipation, some pelvic pain and I woke up 4 times during the night to empty my bladder. He said this indicated there was a problem with the back ligaments of the vagina.

The nurse then drew the curtains and helped me onto the examination couch. She explained that the doctor would examine me internally to see which areas of my vagina were damaged, front, middle, or back.

During the examination, the doctor asked me to cough and confirmed that I leaked urine (stress incontinence). He then gently pressed upwards with an instrument on that part of the vagina just behind the pubic bone and asked me to cough again. I noticed that this prevented urine leakage. He said it proved that

医生解释说,这些问卷的目的是发现异常的症状,并推测阴道的哪些部分受到了损伤。他给我看了下面的示意图,说:

"不要过分注重细节,只要看这3列,标记的地方就是问题所在。您会看到3个潜在的损伤区域:前部、中部和后部,每个区域都有特定的症状和脱垂器官。"

然后他告诉我,脱垂是膀胱、子宫或肠道引起的阴道内块物。盆底松弛是可以修复的。

他让我参考诊断图示再次回答问卷。

例如,问卷的第一个问题:*"您咳嗽时有漏尿吗?"*

我回答"是"。医生在"压力性尿失禁"栏打了勾,解释说我的阴道前部韧带有问题。

接下来的问卷中我回答说,"我感觉膀胱不能完全排空,有尿急、便秘、盆腔疼痛,并且夜间起床排尿4次。"他说,这表明我的阴道后部韧带也有问题。

护士拉上窗帘,协助我上了检查床。她解释说医生要给我做内诊,以明确阴道的哪些部位受损,是前部、中部还是后部。

检查时,医生让我咳嗽并确认我有漏尿(压力性尿失禁)。然后,他用器械在耻骨后方的阴道部分轻轻上抬,再次让我咳嗽。我注意到这样子可以阻止尿液漏出。他说这证明了我的前部韧带有损伤。然后他让我"用力向下屏气"(加压),判断是否有脱垂。

医生和我讨论了初步检查的发现,说需要进一步检查来确定问题的严重性。这些检查包括:超声检查、24小时排尿日记、24小时尿垫试验和尿动力学检查。护士给了我相关知识的小册子,并做了详细解释。

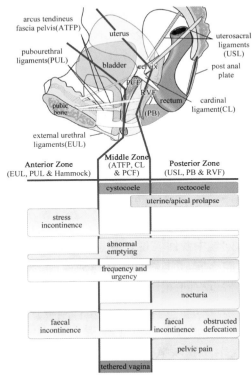

Fig 9 - 1 The Diagnostic Diagram is used by some doctors to explain
the relationship of damaged ligaments to prolapse and
symptoms. The doctor ticks the symptoms and these give a
visual guide as to which ligaments have been damaged. The
height of the column indicates the likelihood of the symptom
occurring in that part of the vagina.

Pubourethral Ligament (PUL)

Hammock

Extrernal Urethral Ligament (EUL)

Pubocervical fascia (PCF)

Cardinal Ligament/cervical ring

Arcus Tendineus Fascia Pelvis (ATFP)

Uterosacral Ligament (USL)

Rectovaginal fascia (RVF)

Perineal body (PB)

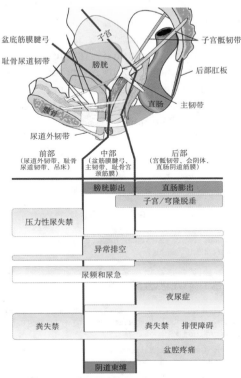

图9-1 诊断图示 被一些医生用来解释盆底韧带损伤与症状和脱垂的关系。医生标记症状，根据图示可以直观地看到哪些韧带发生了损伤。图示中横柱高度代表这部分阴道出现某个症状的概率

耻骨尿道韧带(pubourethral ligament，PUL)

吊床(hammock)

尿道外韧带(exrernal urethral ligament，EUL)

耻骨宫颈筋膜(pubocervical fascia，PCF)

主韧带/宫颈环[cardinal ligament(CL)/cervical ring]

盆筋膜腱弓(arcus tendineus fascia pelvis，ATFP)

宫骶韧带(uterosacral ligament，USL)

直肠阴道筋膜(rectovaginal fascia，RVF)

会阴体(perineal body，PB)

my front ligament was damaged. He then asked me to 'push down into my bottom' (strain), so he could see if I had a prolapse.

The doctor discussed the preliminary findings and said I needed further tests to ascertain how serious my problem was. These tests included ultrasound, a 24 hour urinary diary, a 24 hour pad test and urodynamics testing. I was given pamphlets and further detailed explanations by the nurse.

Contents of the Twenty Four Hour Diary pamphlet:

TWENTY FOUR HOUR DIARY

The diary records your volume intake, output wet episodes, and it collects your history.

TWENTY FOUR HOUR: PAD TEST

This is an important test, as it gives us an accurate assessment of how much urine leaks in an uncontrolled way during a 24 hour period.

1. One vitamin B tablet is taken just before the test begins, to colour your urine dark yellow.

2. You commence the pad test and the diary the day before so the 24 hours is complete a few hours before your appointment.

Set aside one dry menstrual pad for weighing by the nurse. It is important that you wear a pad at all times for 24 hours before your appointment. Each time you feel your pad is wet, you place it into the sealed plastic bag provided by the clinic, and replace it with a dry pad.

24 小时排尿日记小册子的内容:

24 小时排尿日记

排尿日记作为病史收集,记录您的摄水量和漏尿发作次数。

24 小时尿垫试验

这是一项重要的试验,能准确地评估 24 小时内的不自主漏尿量。

1. 在检查开始前服用一片维生素 B 药片,让尿液变成深黄色。

2. 在就诊前几个小时,完成 24 小时排尿日记和尿垫试验。

预留一个干燥的卫生巾,由护士称重。重要的是,在就诊前的 24 小时内,您应始终佩戴卫生巾。每次感到卫生巾潮湿时,请将其放入诊所提供的密封塑料袋中,更换干燥的卫生巾。

Contents of the Urodynamic testing pamphlet:

URODYNAMIC TESTING

Urodynamics measures bladder pressures. During Urodynamic testing, we measure the amount of urine loss during 10 coughs. Then a small 2mm diameter pressure measuring device is inserted into the urethra to measure what happens during various manoeuvres. A small telescopic instrument is inserted into the urethra to examine the inside of your bladder, and to test the strength of your closure muscles.

At the end of this testing, you will sit on a commode and empty your bladder.

Total time for Urodynamic testing is approximately 20 to 30 minutes.

ON RETURNING HOME FROM URODYNAMIC TESTING

Please remember your body has been though a lot today. Rest and drink plenty of fluids to flush and minimize any discomfort on urinating. If a small amount of discomfort or slight spotting of blood is noticed, this can be normal after this test, and a warm bath often helps. An Aspirin/Panadol may be taken if required. Please follow the directions on the package.

My Second Consultation

When I arrived again at the clinic for further testing. I handed the nurse my 24 hours urinary diary and the plastic bag containing all the wet pads for the past 24 hours. She then asked me to empty my bladder. I was taken into a special room for urodynamics. I found the urodynamics testing reasonably comfortable. I stood up. A pad was placed in my briefs and I coughed 10 times to assess the severity of my stress incontinence. The nurse weighed the pad to measure how much urine I lost during coughing. The ultrasound examination was quite painless. An ultrasound probe was placed outside my vagina. A picture was taken at rest. I was then asked to cough and then to strain downwards. I was able to observe how my

尿动力学检查小册子的内容:

尿动力学检查

尿动力学测查的是膀胱压力。在尿动力学检查中,我们记录 10 次咳嗽时的漏尿量,然后将一个直径 2 mm 的测压装置放入尿道,测量各种动作时的压力情况。然后将一个小型可伸缩装置插入尿道,检查膀胱内部情况,并检测闭合尿道的肌肉强度。

检查结束后,您将坐在一个马桶上排尿。

尿动力学检查的总时间为 20~30 分钟。

做完尿动力学检查回家后

请记住,今天您的身体经历了很多。要注意休息并大量饮水,以冲洗尿路并减少排尿时的不适。如果检查后出现轻微不适或少量出血,大多是正常的,洗个热水澡通常会有帮助。必要时可服用阿司匹林/扑热息痛,请按照药品包装上的说明服用。

我的第二次就诊

再次到诊所做进一步检查时,我将 24h 排尿日记和装着过去 24h 所有湿卫生巾的塑料袋交给了护士。她让我去排空膀胱,把我带到一个专门的尿动力学检查室。尿动力学检查还算舒服。我保持站立的姿势,一块护垫衬在内裤里,咳嗽 10 次以评估尿失禁的严重程度。护士称量了那块护垫来评估我在咳嗽时的漏尿量。超声检查也毫无痛苦,探头放置在阴道口外面。静息状态下先采集一幅图像,然后咳嗽,随即用力增加腹压向下屏气。在向下用力时,我看到膀胱变成了漏斗状,甚至看到尿液漏出来了。然后我将尿液排到一个特殊的容器里,测量尿流率

bladder went into the shape of a funnel when I pushed downwards. I even saw the urine leaking out. I then emptied my bladder into a special pan to measure the rate of urine flow and time taken to empty. When I had finished, the ultrasound measured how much urine remained in my bladder. This is known as the residual urine. When all the testing was complete, I was taken to see the doctor. The doctor reviewed all the results and discussed them with me, one by one: the urinary diary, the 24 hours pad test, the 10 cough test, the ultrasound and the urodynamics. He referred to a diagram of the vagina and bladder and pointed out which ligaments were damaged. I anxiously asked the doctor how serious my problem was and what he thought was the best way to fix me.

The doctor said that the pad test results indicated that pelvic floor exercises were unlikely to be successful and I would most likely require surgery to reinforce the front and back ligaments. He gave me some explanatory pamphlets, told me to ring if I had any questions and to return at a later date should I decide to proceed with the surgery.

I discussed the matter with my husband and returned at a later date.

Consent for Surgery

The doctor brought out a consent form to which he referred as he explained the risks and benefits of the surgery that was proposed and the possible complications. He encouraged me to ask any questions which came to mind during the consent process. Referring to the form again, he proceeded to explain other treatment options, including alternative surgical procedures and the risks and benefits thereof. He used a printed diagram and a hand drawing to illustrate how he proposed to strengthen the damaged front and back ligaments by inserting short tapes. He said that the operation was reasonably painless and could be done with a very short hospital stay. The main problem requiring a longer stay was inability to pass urine immediately after surgery. This was uncommon. If this happened, it was usually temporary and could require a catheter for a few days.

I was then asked to read the consent form and we discussed each item on it more fully, including the complications of the procedure proposed, other options for treatment and why he thought these were not suitable for me.

和排空时间,这些步骤结束后,用超声测量膀胱中残留的尿量,这被称为残余尿(residual urine)。

所有检查完成后,我被带去见医生。医生认真地看了所有的检查结果,并和我一起逐个讨论:排尿日记、24 小时尿垫试验、10 次咳嗽试验,超声和尿动力学检查。他参考了阴道和膀胱关系的图示,指出哪些韧带存在损伤。我焦急地询问医生目前问题的严重程度,而他考虑的是最佳的修复治疗方案。

医生说,尿垫试验表明盆底训练的成功率不高,很有可能需要通过手术来加强前部和后部韧带。他给了我一些答疑的小册子,表示如果有任何疑问可以来电咨询。如果我决定继续手术的话,过段时间来复诊。

我和丈夫讨论了这件事情,后来去复诊了。

手术知情同意

医生拿出了一份手术知情同意书,他向我解释手术可能的风险和益处,以及可能出现的并发症。在签署知情同意书的过程中,医生鼓励我提出所有想到的问题。再次回到手术知情同意书时,他接着向我解释其他治疗方案,包括替代的手术方案及其风险和获益。此外,医生还用打印的诊断图示和手绘图向我说明,如何通过置入短吊带来加固前部和后部损伤的韧带。他说这个手术是基本无痛的,住院时间很短。需要延长住院时间的主要原因是手术后无法即时排尿,但这种情况很罕见,如果发生了这种情况,通常都是暂时的,可能需要留置导尿一段时间来恢复。

阅读了手术知情同意书后,我们共同全面讨论了上面的每一个条目,包括:所建议手术的并发症、其他可供选择的治疗方案以及这些方案不适合我的原因。

What to Do After Discharge from the Hospital

Because of the risk of sutures tearing out, for at least 6 weeks postoperatively I was told not do any heavy lifting, exercise, squatting, straining or vaginal intercourse. I could, however, drive my car after a few days, do some shopping and even go to work. I should avoid opening my legs or bending down without bending my knees. I should keep my legs together and swing both knees sideways when getting in and out of a car.

I was told that patients usually experience very little pain postoperatively but if there was severe pain, I should contact the doctor immediately.

I could expect some bleeding of dark blood for a few days postoperatively but not to worry about this. If the bleeding was excessive in the first 48 hours and especially if there were clots, I must contact the doctor immediately.

If I had a temperature postoperatively, I must contact the doctor immediately, as I may have an infection. The nurse would give me pamphlets. I was to read the pamphlets carefully, as they contained all the relevant information relating to my procedure.

Because I was to spend only one day in hospital, I had to see the doctor a week after the procedure.

At the end of the consent process, I was asked if I understood what was involved in the surgical procedure and if I had any questions. I then signed the Consent form which the doctor witnessed and dated.

The doctor wrote out a form for some pre-operative blood tests and for a swab taken from the vagina to check for bacteria which could possibly cause infection after the surgery. I was given a suppository to be taken the night before surgery to empty my bowel and a prescription for antibiotic tablets, also to be taken the night before surgery.

The nurse then ushered me to the secretary where I was given further instructions, an appointment to see my anaesthetist, more specific information about my surgery and further information pamphlets. I was asked to cease all aspirin 10 days before surgery and to bring along a list of my current medications when I visited the anaesthetist.

出院后该做些什么?

由于存在术后缝线撕脱的风险,我被告知在术后至少 6 周内不能做任何搬运重物、运动、下蹲、向下用力或阴道性交。不过,几天后我就可以开车、购物,甚至上班。我应该避免张开双腿或者不弯曲膝盖的弯腰动作。上下车时,我应该保持双腿并拢,两个膝盖摆向同一侧。

我被告知,术后仅有轻微的疼痛。一旦出现剧烈疼痛,应立即联系医生。

术后几天,可能会有少量暗红色出血,但无须担心。如果术后 48 小时内出血很多,尤其是有血块,必须立即联系医生。

如果术后出现体温升高,我必须立即联系医生,因为可能是感染了。护士给我一些小册子,要我仔细阅读这些小册子,因为它们包含了所有与手术相关的信息。由于我只住院一天,所以术后 1 周必须去诊所随访。

知情同意过程的最后,医生询问我是否理解了手术过程涉及的所有内容以及是否还有疑问。最后,在医生见证下我签署了知情同意书,并注明了日期。

医生填了一份表格,罗列了一些术前血液检查结果,以及阴道拭子检测是否存在可能导致术后感染的细菌。医生给我开了一枚栓剂用于手术前一天晚上排空肠道;还有抗生素片剂,也在手术前一天晚上服用。

然后,护士把我带到诊所秘书那里,得到了更进一步的指导。预约了见麻醉师的时间,获得了更多关于手术的具体信息和包含更多信息的小册子。手术前 10 天应停止服用阿司匹林,在与麻醉师见面时须携带目前服用的药物清单。

An example of the pre-operative information pamphlet given to me.

PRE-OPERATIVE INFORMATION

Fasting requirements

If surgery is to be performed on the morning list then you should have nothing to eat, drink or smoke from midnight the night before. If the operation is to be performed on the afternoon list then it is permissible to have a light breakfast that morning before 7.00am and nothing more to eat, drink or smoke before your operation.

A light breakfast consists of:

A slice of toast, cup of tea/coffee.

or

Half a bowl of cereal, cup of tea/coffee.

You are requested to trim any long hairs around your pubic area.

Notify Dr P...... Should you Develop a cough or cold before the operation or your menstrual cycle has commenced.

Please bring a packet of sanitary pads with you to hospital with your own night attire and toiletries.

我拿到的术前宣教小册子的样张：

术前信息

禁食要求

　　如果手术在上午施行，从前一天午夜开始您就什么都不能吃、不能喝，也不能抽烟。如果手术在下午施行，允许在早上7点之前少量进食早餐，但手术前不能吃、不能喝，也不能抽烟。

　　简单的早餐包括：

　　一片吐司，一杯茶/咖啡

　　或

　　半碗麦片粥，一杯茶/咖啡。

　　您要将阴阜周围区域的阴毛修剪干净。如果手术前出现咳嗽或感冒，或者月经来潮，应当告知医生。

　　请携带一包卫生巾和您自己的睡衣和洗漱用品到医院。

An example of the post-operative information pamphlet given to me.

First 12 to 24 hours post-operatively

You will wake up in the post-operative anaesthetic recovery room within the theatre area. You may have an oxygen mask fitted comfortably over your mouth and nose. There may be an intra-venous "drip" (IV) needle in your arm.

Analgesic medication will be prescribed to prevent and post-operative pain. The pain is usually minimal. You may have has a spinal anaesthetic, in which case your legs and areas from the waist down may be numb the first few hours until the spinal anaesthetic wears off. Some patients experience nausea and may vomit during the first few hours after returning from the ward. Medication to counteract nausea and vomiting is routinely prescribed during your operation.

The nursing staff will measure your urine during the first 12 to 24 hours pots-operatively to watch for any retention (build-up of urine in your bladder). If you are not passing enough urine, the nursing staff may have to pass a small "in-out" catheter to check your bladder. This catheter does not remain in your bladder.

我拿到的术后宣教小册子的样张：

术后 12～24 小时

您将在手术室的麻醉复苏区域醒来。嘴巴和鼻子上舒适地罩着一个氧气面罩，手臂上可能有静脉留置针。

术后将使用镇痛药物来缓解疼痛。疼痛通常都非常轻微。如果您是脊椎麻醉，术后数小时内会有双腿和腰部以下区域的麻木感，直到麻醉效果退去。有些患者刚回到病房的数小时会有恶心，甚至呕吐。通常，术中会用药物抑制恶心、呕吐等反应。

术后的 12～24 小时，护理人员会记录您的尿量，以观察是否有尿潴留（尿液积聚在膀胱中）。如果您的尿量不足，护理人员可能会用一个"由内而外"的小导管来检查您的膀胱，该导管不会留置在膀胱中。

VAGINAL REPAIR

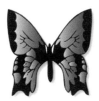

Issued by:
The Kvinno Centre

6. FOLLOW-UP

An initial appointment should be made one week after the operation, or earlier if there is a problem. There is a further follow-up at 6 weeks. There may be some vaginal bleeding in the first few days after the operation. You should be able to pass urine normally. For the first few days, you may experience some urgency i.e. A desire to pass urine frequently. This could be a result of the catheter used at the operation or due to swelling around the sutures.

7. RESULTS OF THE OPERATION

The results of any operation cannot be guaranteed, but if you are careful, the results are normally excellent. However, unlike other types of vaginal repair operations, there should be cure of the prolapse with minimal discomfort and a rapid return to normal activities because the vaginal skin is not excised. If there is no improvement it is due to the sutures tearing out of damaged tissues, but because the vaginal is not excised the operation can be easily adjusted later to improve results.

阴道修复

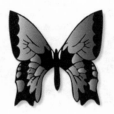

Kvinno 中心发行

6. 随访

初次随访在术后一周进行，如果期间有问题可以提前。术后 6 周第二次复诊。术后几天内可能会有少量阴道出血。您可以正常地排尿。在刚开始的几天，您可能会觉得尿急（一种需要频繁排尿的症状）。这可能是由于手术时使用导尿管或缝线周围的水肿所致。

7. 手术效果

任何手术都无法保证百分百成功，但如果您足够小心，一般效果都很好。与其他阴道修复手术不同的是，这个手术并不切除阴道黏膜，因此治愈脱垂所经历的痛苦更小，恢复到日常生活的速度也更快。如果症状没有改善，可能是因为受损的组织缝线撕脱了。但是因为没有切除阴道黏膜，就很容易再次手术调整以提高疗效。

8. COMPLICATIONS

Complications are rare, but it must be understood and accepted that these can occur. The complications that can occur include, but are not limited to:

a) Infection – there may be a simple infection of the urine or pelvis requiring antibiotics alone. However, a pelvic abscess could develop requiring drainage.

b) Haemorrhage – this is extremely rare, but is watched postoperatively.

c) Retention of Urine – this is rare, but if it did occur, a catheter would need to be inserted.

d) Injury to Bladder – During dissection, an incision may be made in the bladder. This would be repaired and a catheter inserted.

e) Injury to Ureter – the ureter which brings urine from the kidney to the bladder may be kinked or tied. This could cause pain in the kidney and possible fistula formation, and would require an abdominal operation to correct and reimplant it into the bladder.

f) Injury to Bowel – if there is an enterocoele, the bowel could be caught by a suture, and this would require an abdominal incision to correct.

g) Deep Venous Thrombosis – a possible complication of any surgery, but much less likely with this type of operation where you are mobilized almost immediately.

It must be emphasized that complications are extremely rare with this type of surgery, and most of the above have not yet been encountered.

162

8. 并发症

并发症很少见,但必须理解并接受并发症是有可能发生的。可能发生的并发症包括但不限于以下几项:

a)感染——可能是简单的尿路或者盆腔感染,只需应用抗生素治疗,也有可能发展为盆腔脓肿而需要手术引流。

b)大出血——很少见,但术后也曾发生过。

c)尿潴留——少见,一旦出现需要使用导尿管。

d)膀胱损伤——在手术分离过程中,可能损伤膀胱,需要手术修补和留置导尿。

e)输尿管损伤——将尿液从肾脏送到膀胱的输尿管可能发生扭曲或被缝扎,会引起肾区疼痛或者输尿管瘘,需要经腹手术纠正,将其重新置入膀胱中。

f)肠道损伤——如果合并肠疝,手术中可能会缝住肠管从而造成损伤,需要经腹手术修补。

g)深静脉血栓形成——所有手术都可能发生的并发症,但这种类型的手术后可以立即活动,几乎很少发生。

必须强调的是,这种类型的手术并发症很少发生,而上述情况中的大多数尚未遇到过。

Comment

An example of the pamphlet for vaginal repair. Similar pamphlets are given for the other operations. The complications listed are rare but it is important to fully inform the patient.

A Successful Result

My operation went well. I had some pain initially, mainly from the sutures but this improved after the sutures were removed prior to discharge from hospital. I saw the doctor a week after surgery and again at 6 weeks for a more comprehensive review. He used my questionnaire form as a reference point to check my symptoms. My stress incontinence was cured. I was only getting up once a night to go to the toilet. I still had some feelings of urgency but very rarely wet now. My pelvic pain was still present but I esti-mated it was at least 90% improved. I was emptying better and the ultrasound showed very little urine remained in the bladder after I had emptied it. The doctor asked me to return in 3 months for further follow-up.

点评

阴道修复手术宣教小册子是一个例子。其他的手术也有类似的宣教手册。列出的手术并发症都很少见，但需要充分告知患者。

满意的结果

我的手术进展顺利。最初有些疼痛，主要来自缝线处，出院前拆除缝线后，疼痛有所缓解。术后 1 周初次复诊，术后 6 周进行了更全面的检查。医生用我的问卷调查表作为参考，核对症状。压力性尿失禁已经治愈，每晚只需上一次厕所。我仍然觉得有点尿急，但已很少漏尿。盆腔疼痛仍然存在，但自我感觉已经改善了 90％。膀胱排空得到改善，超声检查提示排尿后膀胱的残余尿很少。医生要求我 3 个月后做进一步的随访。

（上海交通大学医学院附属第六人民医院妇产科，李洁 译，薛卓维 校）

165

CHAPTER 10   Summary—
"What do I do—where do I go?"

Summary and Conclusions

The methods discussed in this book offer hope and help for the millions of women who are enduring the pain, both physical and psychological, associated with bladder or bowel incontinence and chronic pelvic pain. There is no need to suffer in silence and no need to accept the mentally debilitating statements that there is no possible cure for symptoms such as chronic pelvic pain, nocturia, urgency, abnormal emptying even many cases of faecal incontinence. We emphasize that many of these symptoms can be cured or significantly improved by strengthening damaged ligaments either with time efficient muscle exercises or by repairing them surgically with the minimally invasive operations discussed in this book.

You, too, may be helped, as were the many women who attended our clinic. Have the courage to speak to your doctor about the problems you are experiencing. Use the information in this book to empower you towards achieving a better quality of life. Take the book along to your doctor and discuss one of the histories relevant to your condition. The science is known and substantially proven. It is a matter of the physician becoming informed about these innovative methods.

As regards the science, fortunately, the thinking which has dominated treatment for the last 100 years is beginning to change.

A major factor in this change is the scientific questioning of urodynamics (bladder pressure measurement) as a guide to treatment. Urodynamic assessment forms the very cornerstone of traditional thinking. If a patient has certain urodynamic findings, urgency or nocturia, surgery is said not to be an option. This is not only incorrect, it is tragic, as millions of women are condemned to a lifetime of misery by the failure of this method.

第十章　总结

——我该做什么？　我该去哪里就诊？

总结与讨论

本书讨论的方法为数百万女性患者提供了希望和帮助，这些女性在身心上都忍受着与尿失禁或粪失禁以及慢性盆腔疼痛相关的痛苦。无须默默忍受，也无须被迫接受慢性盆腔痛、夜尿症、尿急、排空异常甚至粪失禁等症状都无法治愈的无知言论。我们主张通过及时有效的盆底肌肉训练来加强受损的韧带，或者通过本书中讨论的微创手术进行手术修复，这样就可以治愈或显著改善以上症状。

您也能像在我们诊所就诊的许多女性朋友一样得到帮助。请勇敢地与您的医生讲述您所面临的问题。本书中的相关信息可以帮助您提高生活质量。您可以将本书随身带给医生，和他讨论其中与您病情相关的病史。本书中的知识已发展得相对成熟，并且已得到了充分证明。这本书也有助于医生了解这些创新的方法。

比较幸运的是，就盆底这一亚学科而言，过去100年来主导治疗的思想正在开始改变。引起这种变化的主要因素是对将尿动力学检查（膀胱压力测量）作为治疗指导的科学质疑。尿动力学评估是传统治疗思维的基础。过去认为，如果患者尿动力学检查发现异常，有尿急或夜尿症，则不能选择手术。这不仅是不正确的，而且是可悲的，因为这种评估结果的错误，使数百万妇女遭受了一生的痛苦。

Self Diagnosis

Self Diagnosis is not advisable even for someone medically trained! However, within the context of information, it is useful to understand the Diagnostic Diagram, Fig 10 − 1, which allows a coarse estimate of the origins of symptoms. At a glance, you can see which ligaments may be causing the particular problem you may be experiencing. Simply go to the top of each column in turn and scan down.

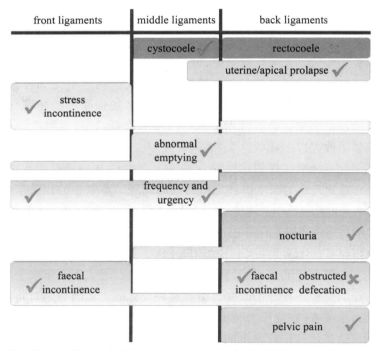

Fig 10 − 1   Diagnostic Diagram -the causal relationship between damaged ligaments, prolapse and symptoms. Read vertically from top to bottom for each ligament.

自我诊断

即使是经过医学培训的人,也不建议进行自我诊断! 然而,医学背景有助于理解以下诊断图示(见图 10 - 1)。该图示可以粗略地推断引起症状的源头,哪些韧带损伤引起您的特定问题一目了然。您只需依次从每一列的顶部向下浏览即可。

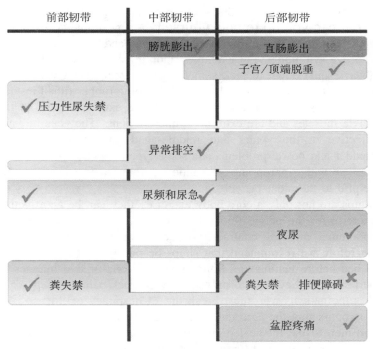

图 10 - 1　诊断图示——韧带损伤、脱垂和症状之间的因果关系。从上到下垂直分析每条韧带

The "tampon test"

This is a test, not a treatment. It can confirm if a loose back ligament may be causing the symptoms. It should be carried out with a bladder which is sufficiently full for symptoms to be present.

Insert one large or two standard tampons together as far as possible into the back part of the vagina. If the pain or urge symptoms are relieved, this is a good indication that loose ligaments may be causing the problem and that the symptoms are potentially curable.

What can you do to help yourself? A few simple changes to a daily routine will improve muscle toning and may significantly improve symptoms. For example, adopting a "squatting culture" : always squat down to pick something up rather than bend down; squat while doing routine chores. Sitting on a rubber fitball instead of a chair at work or watching TV. These exercises train all the pelvic muscles and are extremely time efficient. They can be very effective in the young and middle-aged patient in improving bladder and bowel problems and some types of pelvic pain. When applied with appropriate precautions, they may sometimes be helpful to the older patient.

Situps are not only a core body exercise, they can be an effective exercise for the pelvic floor. It is not well known that when the abdominal muscles contract, so do the pelvic floor muscles. Therefore we recommend that situps be performed every morning in bed before getting up. Situps take only one or two minutes to perform and they help to prevent chronic back pain.

It is the patients who must break the "Conspiracy of Silence" by communicating the core messages of this book, first to each other and then to the medical profession, because the many conditions hither to considered incurable, can indeed be cured or improved in a high percentage of cases.

"卫生棉条试验"

这是一种试验，而不是治疗。它可以帮助确认松弛的后部韧带是否引起了相关症状。为了更好地诱发症状，试验应在膀胱充盈的情况下进行。

将一个大号或两个标准大小的卫生棉条尽可能塞入阴道后部。如果疼痛或尿急症状得到缓解，则表明该症状是由后部韧带松弛引起的，这些症状有可能被治愈。

您能做些什么来帮助自己呢？ 日常生活的一些简单改变会使肌肉更有力量，并可能显著地改善症状。例如，采用"蹲式文化"：总是蹲下来捡东西而不是弯腰；蹲着做日常家务。坐在橡胶健身球而不是椅子上工作或看电视。这些练习可以锻炼所有的盆底肌肉，并且非常省时高效。这种锻炼方法在中青年患者中可以非常有效地改善膀胱和直肠问题以及某些类型的盆腔疼痛。如果采取适当的预防措施，也可能对年长的患者有所帮助。

仰卧起坐不仅是一项躯干部位的训练，也可以成为一种有效的盆底训练方法。鲜为人知的是，当腹部肌肉收缩时，骨盆底肌肉也会随之收缩。因此，我们建议每天早晨起床前进行仰卧起坐锻炼。仰卧起坐仅需一两分钟即可完成，并且有助于预防慢性背部疼痛。

首先，患者通过彼此交流本书的核心信息，然后与医生进行沟通，从而打破"缄默的密约"，因为许多目前认为无法治愈的疾病，很大比例上是可以被治愈或改善的。

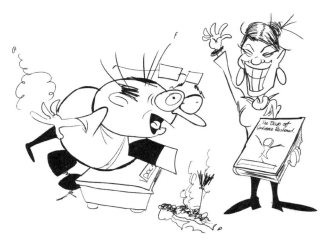

Fig 10 – 2   Look, Doc, this is what my problem is

Surgery—where do I go? If the exercises fail, what next? How does one empower a woman as regards surgery? The first step is information. The second step is how she uses that information.

It is a simple matter for a reader to bring the book to her doctor to discuss a relevant case history from chapters 4,5 or 6. The doctor will know about the midurethral sling surgical procedure (TVT), which cures urinary stress incontinence in up to 90% of patients by strengthening the front ligaments with an implanted tape, as this operation is almost universal. What is not well known is that this operation (the TVT) is applicable to many other conditions besides stress incontinence, as detailed in the Chapter 4 stories.

What is also not well understood, is that the back ligaments, Chapter 6, are a major cause of incapacitating symptoms such as urgency, nocturia, inability to empty properly, some types of chronic pelvic pain and even bowel symptoms. Traditional operations, some extremely simple, already exist which can

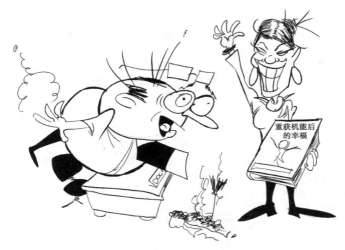

图 10 - 2　快看,医生,这就是我的问题

　　手术——我该何去何从?　如果盆底训练失败,下一步该怎么办? 如何在手术方面赋予女性权力? 第一步是信息,第二步是她如何使用该信息。

　　对于读者来说,将本书带到医生那里并与之讨论第四、第五或第六章中的相关病例是很简便的。医生将了解有关尿道中段悬吊手术(TVT)的信息,该手术通过置入吊带加强前部韧带,可治愈 90% 的压力性尿失禁患者,目前这种手术方式几乎是普遍开展的。很多人并不知道,该手术(TVT)除压力性尿失禁外还适用于治疗许多其他问题,具体内容见本书第四章所述。

　　目前还不是很清楚,后部韧带是否是导致失能症状的主要原因,例如尿急、夜尿、排空异常、某些类型的慢性盆腔疼痛,甚至肠道症状等(如本书第六章所述)。目前仍在采用的传统手术

tighten the back ligaments*, albeit somewhat less successfully than the TFS tape reinforcement techniques used in the stories in this book. These are comprehensively described in Chapter 4 of the medical textbook, "*The Female Pelvic Floor*", 3rd Edition, by PEP Petros, Springer Heidelberg, 2010 and also, in scientific papers available at www. integraltheory. org. The textbook greatly expands on the information in this book and provides references to hundreds of scientific papers also by other authors on various aspects of this system of care as further background and proof.

It is a matter of significant concern to the authors that even this most simple of methods is unknown to many physicians. At present, women with such symptoms are told no help is possible and they have to live with their condition, a cruel contribution to the passive conspiracy of silence. These women, some as young as 30 or 40 are condemned to a lifetime of pain, embarrassment, erosion of self-confidence and self-esteem. This book was written especially to empower such women, so they can become the catalyst for the change in thinking required to bring help and hope to conditions which are not only potentially curable, but curable with minimally invasive methods.

Scientific Data and specialists in this method

The Medical profession (correctly so), requires scientific data published in peer review journals, before making any decisions to explore new treatment methods. The table presented below is from but one of many published papers on the Integral System. It

---

* The simplest possible operation to tighten the back ligaments is safe and minimally invasive. It can be performed even under local anaesthesia by making a small horizontal incision 3 − 4 cm behind the cervix and tightening the back ligaments with normal sutures. This minor operation produced the following cure of symptoms at 3 months: urge incontinence, 55%; abnormal emptying, 60%; pelvic pain, 75%; pain on deep penetration on intercourse, 68%, with an equivalent cure rate for nocturia (getting up at night to pass urine). A much higher cure rate for such symptoms over a longer period is possible using a thin strip of tape to strengthen the back ligaments.

中,有些手术方式非常简单,可以有效地紧缩后部韧带*,尽管其成功率不如本书举例中所使用的 TFS 吊带加强方式。在 PEP Petros 所著的《女性骨盆底》第三版(2010 年)的第四章中对此进行了全面描述,相关论文也可在 www. integraltheory. org 网站上获取。该教材极大地丰富了本书中的内容,并提供了数百篇由其他作者所著、有关该系统各个方面的科学论文作为参考,以及进一步研究的背景和证据。

作者非常关注的问题是,许多医生并不了解这些最简单的方法。目前,患有此类症状的很多妇女被告知不能提供任何有效的帮助给她们,她们必须伴随该症状一直生活下去,此类消极现象是我们称为"缄默的密约"的重要体现。这些妇女,有些年仅 30 或 40 多岁,她们将遭受一生的痛苦、尴尬以及自信心和自尊心的日渐消磨。编写本书的一个重要目的是为了赋予这些妇女权力,并使她们成为改变传统思维方式的催化剂,给那些不仅可能被治愈甚至可以通过微创方法治愈的患者带去帮助和希望。

应用此疗法的科学数据和专家

在做出任何探索新治疗方法的决定之前,医学界(非常正确)要求在同行评议的期刊上发表科学数据。下表来自于已发表的众多关于"整体理论系统"的论文中的一篇。它总结了与本

---

* 这种最简单的紧缩后部韧带的手术是安全并且微创的。即使在局部麻醉下,也可以通过在子宫颈后方 3~4 cm 处做一个水平的小切口,并用常规缝合线拉紧后部韧带。此手术在术后 3 个月时可治愈以下症状:55% 的急迫性尿失禁;60% 的排空异常;75% 的盆腔疼痛;68% 的深部性交疼痛,68% 的夜尿症(夜间起床排尿)。此外,使用较细的吊带来加固后部韧带,可以在更长的时间内获得更高的治愈率。

summarizes information relevant to the stories in this book.

Table 10-1 Symptom Outcome - 67 patients.

Symptom change with surgery			% cure in brackets		
Faecal incontinence	Frequency > 10/Day	Nocturia > 2/night	Urge incontinence > 2/day	Abnormal emptying	Pelvic pain
Australia					
$n = 23$	$n = 27$	$n = 47$	$n = 36$	$n = 53$	$n = 46$
(87%)	(63%)	(83%)	(78%)	(73%)	(86%)
$P \leq 0.005$	$P \leq 0.005$	$P \leq 0.005$	$P \leq 0.005$	$P \leq 0.005$	$P \leq 0.005$
Japan 336 patients					
$n = 52$	$n = 179$	$n = 129$	$n = 171$	NA	$n = 76$
(82.7%)	(84.9%)	(60.5%)	(91.2%)	NA	(71.1%)

© 2013 The Authors
ANZJOG © 2013 The Royal Australian and New Zealand College of Obstetricians and Gynaecologists

325

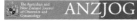

Medical data from 403 patients with "incurable" symptoms after a TFS posterior sling was inserted to strengthen the back ligaments of the vagina

The top row describes the symptoms. "n" refers to the number of cases for each symptom.
The percentage in brackets on the bottom line refers to the percentage of patients who were cured by the operation in each symptom.

These data, 403 cases from two different centres, are only one of many examples which confirm that many conditions that were previously considered as being incurable—for example, fecal incontinence, nocturia (getting up at night to pass urine), urge incontinence (unable to control the bladder), chronic low abdominal or pelvic pain, frequency (going frequently) , inability to empty the bladder properly—were cured or very significantly improved by repairing the back ligaments of the vagina.
A large selection of original scientific articles on the topics of this book are available on www. integraltheory. org or on www. pelviperineology. org or by internet search in other scientific journals using keywords such as "Tissue Fixation System", TFS, Integral Theory, posterior sling repair and other words taken from this book.

书病例相关的信息。

表10-1 症状结果——67位患者

| 手术后症状改善 | | | 括号中为治愈比例(%) | | |
粪失禁	尿频 >10次／日	夜尿 >2次／晚	急迫性尿失禁 >2次／日	膀胱排空异常	盆腔疼痛
澳大利亚					
$n=23$	$n=27$	$n=47$	$n=36$	$n=53$	$n=46$
(87%)	(63%)	(83%)	(78%)	(73%)	(86%)
$P \leqslant 0.005$	$P \leqslant 0.005$	$P \leqslant 0.005$	$P \leqslant 0.005$	$P \leqslant 0.005$	$P \leqslant 0.005$
日本[5]336例					
$n=52$	$n=179$	$n=129$	$n=171$	NA	$n=76$
(82.7%)	(84.9%)	(60.5%)	(91.2%)	NA	(71.1%)

The Australian and
New Zealand Journal
of Obstetrics and
Gynaecology

ANZJOG

这些医学数据来自于 403 例被诊断为"不可治愈"症状的患者,她们被置入 TFS 后部吊带以增强阴道后部韧带。

第一行是症状描述。"n"指的是每种症状的病例数。

每行括号中的百分比是指每种症状通过手术治愈的患者百分比。

来自两个不同中心 403 例的病例数据也只是以前被认为无法治愈的许多疾病中的一部分,如粪失禁、夜尿症(夜间起床排尿)、急迫性尿失禁(无法控制膀胱)、慢性下腹部或盆腔疼痛、尿频(频繁发生)、无法正常排空膀胱。目前,这些病例通过修复阴道后方韧带都被治愈或得到了显著改善。

在 www. integraltheory. org 或 www. pelviperineology. org 网站上可以找到关于本书中讨论的大部分原始科学文章,也可以用"Tissue Fixation System"、TFS、Integral Theory、posterior sling repair 及其他本书中的词汇为关键词在科学期刊中检索。

有志于对这些方法进行深入研究的医生可将"Integral

Surgeons specializing in these methods can be located with a standard internet search with key words such Integral System, Integral Theory, Tissue Fixation System.

Copyright permission All the figures and sketches in this book may be freely reproduced without the permission of the authors.

System""Integral Theory""Tissue Fixation System"作为关键词在互联网上进行检索。

版权许可：本书中所有图表和示意图未经作者许可也可以自由复制。

（上海交通大学医学院附属第六人民医院妇产科，刘梦宇　译，薛卓维　校）

GLOSSARY

Abnormal Emptying The bladder cannot empty properly.

Anus The emptying tube for the bowel.

Back ligaments support the uterus (partly) and the back wall of the vagina. Looseness thereof causes prolapsed of the uterus and symptoms of nocturia, urgency, bladder emptying problems and chronic pelvic pain.

Bladder A receptacle for the urine.

Bladder Training used to treat frequency symptoms. The patient is taught is to "hang on" for longer and longer periods so she goes less frequently.

Bladder emptying difficulty Symptoms: slow stream, starting and stopping, dribbling on standing up after emptying, feeling that the bladder has not emptied.

Bowel A receptacle for faeces.

Catheterisation A plastic or rubber tube is placed through the urethra to empty the bladder.

Collagen consists of tightly bound protein rods. It is the fundamental material which gives the body's structures strength. It acts very much like the steel bar in concrete.

Constipation Difficulty in emptying the bowel. The patient usually strains in attempting to do so.

Cystitis means infection in the bladder.

Cystocele A bulge in the front wall of the vagina.

Faecal incontinence Involuntary loss of wind, liquid or solid faeces.

Fistula A channel between bladder or bowel usually to the vagina which causes urine or faeces to leak into the vagina.

Fitball A large round exercise ball used instead of a chair.

术语释义

排空异常：膀胱无法真正排空。

肛门：肠道排空的出口。

后部韧带：支持子宫（部分）和阴道后壁，这些韧带松弛可导致子宫脱垂和夜尿、尿急、膀胱排空问题和慢性盆腔疼痛。

膀胱：储尿的器官。

膀胱训练：用于治疗尿频症状。要求患者憋尿，逐渐延长排尿间歇时间，以减少排尿频次。

膀胱排空困难：症状为尿流慢、间断排尿、排尿后站起时有滴尿，有膀胱排尿不净感。

肠道：容纳粪便的器官。

导尿：将塑料或橡胶管通过尿道放入膀胱以排空尿液。

胶原：由紧密结合的棒状蛋白质组成，是赋予人体结构力量的基本材料，类似混凝土中钢筋的作用。

便秘：排便困难，患者通常需用力排便。

膀胱炎：膀胱内的感染。

膀胱膨出：阴道前壁的凸出。

粪失禁：不自主地排气、排稀便或成形的粪便。

瘘：通常指膀胱或肠管与阴道间的通道，可导致尿液或粪便漏入阴道。

健身球：替代椅子，用于训练的大圆球。

Frequency Goes to the toilet frequently during the day.

Front ligaments suspend the urethra. Looseness thereof causes mainly stress incontinence with or without urgency.

Hormone Replacement Therapy ("HRT') Use of hormones to replace the oestrogen which ceases at the menopause.

Haemorrhage Heavy loss of blood from the uterus.

Hysterectomy is removal of the uterus, either through the tummy (abdominal) or from the vagina (vaginal).

Integral System A method for diagnosing and treating loose ligaments based on the Integral Theory which states that all prolapses and most symptoms of bladder, bowel, chronic pelvic pain are caused by looseness in the vagina or the ligaments (structures) which support it.

Integral Theory states that all prolapses and most symptoms of bladder, bowel chronic pelvic pain are caused by looseness in the vagina or the ligaments (structures) which support it.

Laparoscopy A 1 cm diameter tube is placed inside the abdomen. Prolapse operations can be performed this way.

Ligaments These are cord-like structures which suspend the vagina and the uterus like a suspension bridge. They contain collagen which provides most of the strength.

Macrophages Special white cells which destroy bacteria.

Manchester Repair An old but still good operation for prolapse of the uterus. The middle and back ligaments are shortened and stitched together.

Menopause When a woman's periods cease.

Mesh Reinforcement Surgery for Prolapse Large sheets of polypropylene mesh anywhere from 5 to 8 cm wide and 10 to 15 cm long are placed behind the vagina or inside the abdominal cavity to prevent prolapse of the uterus, bladder or bowel.

Mesh perforation A hole or fistula is made in the bladder or bowel by the mesh.

Middle ligaments suspend the front wall of the vagina and the uterus (partly). Looseness thereof causes cystocele, a bladder lump

尿频：白天频繁地上厕所。

前部韧带：悬吊尿道。这些韧带松弛主要导致压力性尿失禁，伴或不伴尿急。

激素替代治疗(HRT)：使用激素来替代因绝经而停止分泌的雌激素。

大出血：子宫大量出血。

子宫切除术：经腹部或者经阴道切除子宫。

整体理论系统：一种基于整体理论的诊断和治疗韧带松弛的方法，该理论认为所有的脱垂和大多数的膀胱、肠道症状以及慢性盆腔疼痛都是由阴道或其支持韧带(结构)的松弛所引起。

整体理论：该理论认为所有的脱垂和大多数的膀胱、肠道症状以及慢性盆腔疼痛都是由阴道或其支持韧带(结构)的松弛所引起。

腹腔镜：在腹腔放置一根直径1厘米的鞘管，脱垂手术可以通过这种途径施行。

韧带：悬吊起阴道和子宫的类似于悬索桥的索状结构。韧带中的胶原提供了大部分的强度。

巨噬细胞：能消灭细菌的特殊白细胞。

曼彻斯特手术：一种古老而有效的治疗子宫脱垂的手术方式，缩短了中部和后部的韧带，并将它们缝合在一起。

绝经：女性的月经周期终止。

借助网片加强的脱垂手术：在阴道黏膜下或腹腔内放置5～8 cm宽和10～15 cm长的大张聚丙烯网片，以防止子宫、膀胱或肠管脱垂。

网片穿透：网片导致的膀胱或肠管的孔洞或瘘道。

中部韧带：悬吊阴道前壁和子宫(部分)，这些韧带松弛会造成膀胱膨出，即膀胱像块物一样凸向阴道内，伴或不伴尿急及膀胱排空问题。

in the vagina, with or without urgency or bladder emptying problems.

Midstream specimen of urine A sterile container is thrust into the urine stream half-way through when passing urine.

Midurethral sling or TVT An operation to cure urinary stress incontinence (urine loss on coughing). A small strip of polypropylene tape is placed below the midlle part of the urethra.

Minisling A short strip of tape used to strengthen weak ligaments.

Nocturia Gets up at night to pass urine.

Nocturnal Enuresis Wetting the bed at night.

Pelvic pain Dragging pain, often severe, in the lower abdomen, on intercourse, entrance to the vagina or below the urethra.

Pelvic muscles support the vagina, bladder and bowel from below. They also close and open the urethra and anus.

Pelvic floor exercises (Integral System) The pelvic muscles are trained to more efficiently open and close the urethra and anus. These work even when the patient coughs unawares.

Pelvic floor exercises (Kegel) The patients are taught to squeeze upwards. This prevents urine running out. If, however, the patient coughs unawares, she wets.

Pessaries These are fairly large circular rubber or silicone objects placed in the vagina to prevent bladder, bowel or the uterus bulging out of the vagina.

Perineal body (PB) is a firm structure which separates the lower part of the vagina from the back passage. It supports the vagina from below. If this is damaged, the rectum (bowel) may bulge forwards into the vagina. This is called a "rectocele".

Polypropylene A type of plastic used for slings which is very well tolerated in the body.

Prolapse A lump in the vagina caused by bladder (cystocele) uterus (uterine prolapse) or bowel (rectocele) because the ligaments and vaginal tissues are too weak.

Recurrent Cystitis Infection in the bladder which occur again and again.

中段尿样本：在排尿至一半时，用无菌容器采集到的尿液。

尿道中段吊带或 TVT：一种治疗压力性尿失禁（咳嗽时漏尿）的手术。在尿道中段下方放置一小段聚丙烯吊带。

迷你吊带：用来加强薄弱韧带的短吊带。

夜尿症：夜间多次起床排尿。

夜间遗尿：夜晚尿湿床铺。

盆腔疼痛：下腹部、性交时、阴道入口或尿道下方的牵拉痛，常常会很严重。

盆底肌：从下方支持阴道、膀胱和肠管。该肌群也能闭合和开放尿道及肛门。

盆底训练（整体理论系统）：训练骨盆肌肉，使其能更加有效地开放和闭合尿道及肛门。即使患者无意中咳嗽，骨盆肌肉也能发挥以上作用。

盆底训练（凯格尔训练）：指导患者向上收紧盆底肌，可防止漏尿。然而，如果患者在无意中咳嗽，依旧会漏尿。

子宫托：是一系列相当大的圆形的橡胶或硅胶制品，用于放置在阴道内，防止膀胱、肠道或子宫脱出阴道外。

会阴体（PB）：是一种致密结构，将阴道的下段和后方肛管分开，从下方支持阴道。如果会阴体受损，直肠（肠管）可向前突入阴道，称为"直肠膨出"。

聚丙烯：用于制作吊带的塑料材料，人体对其有良好的耐受性。

脱垂：由于韧带和阴道组织支持太弱，造成膀胱（膀胱膨出）、子宫（子宫脱垂）或肠管（直肠膨出）突入阴道引起的块物。

复发性膀胱炎：膀胱内反复发作的感染。

Rectocele A bulge in the back wall of the vagina is called.

Rectum or Bowel A receptacle for faeces.

Relaxin A hormone which loosens the bonds which bind the collagen rods inside the ligaments and the vagina, so these stretch months before labour begins.

Residual Urine Volume The amount retained in the bladder after passing urine.

Robotic Surgery A type of laparoscopy that is performed by remote control by the surgeons who does it via a 3D screen.

Squatting culture Training oneself to always squat down to pick something up instead of bending. This automatically strengthens all the pelvic muscles.

Stress urinary incontinence Urine loss on coughing.

Symptom A warning bell from the brain that something is wrong with some part of the body.

Tethered Vagina Excessive scarring in the vagina from previous surgery. Its defining symptom is sudden massive urine loss immediately on getting out of bed in the morning.

TFS Tissue Fixation System consisting of a polypropylene sling and anchors at both ends, is used to strengthen the loose pelvic ligament and suspend the prolapsed organ.

TVT An operation to cure urinary stress incontinence (urine loss on coughing). A small strip of polypropylene tape is placed below the middle part of the urethra.

Unstable bladder A patient with these symptoms: cannot "hold on" (urgency) goes to the toilet frequently during the day (frequency) or gets up at night to pass urine (nocturia).

Urethra The emptying tube for the bladder.

Urge incontinence Wetting before arrival to the toilet with a feeling of "have to go".

Urodynamics Measure bladder pressures and flow rate on urination.

Uterine prolapse Descent of the uterus into the vagina.

Vulvodynia Pain or burning at the entrance to the vagina.

直肠膨出：阴道后壁的膨出。

直肠或肠管：容纳粪便的脏器。

松弛素：一种能使韧带和阴道内的胶原纤维结合处松弛的激素。它使得韧带和阴道在分娩前数月就得以伸展。

残尿量：排尿后依然留存在膀胱内的尿液量。

机器人手术：一种腹腔镜手术，由外科医生通过 3D 屏幕远程操控完成。

下蹲文化：训练自己总是蹲下来捡东西而不是弯腰捡。这种动作会不自觉地强化所有骨盆肌肉。

压力性尿失禁：咳嗽时有尿液漏出。

症状：大脑发出的一种警示，表示身体某个部位出了问题。

阴道束缚：由于以往手术后阴道形成过度增生的瘢痕造成。典型症状为早晨起床后出现大量漏尿。

组织固定系统（TFS）：由一根吊带和其两端的锚钉组成，用于加强松弛的骨盆韧带，悬吊脱垂的器官。

无张力阴道吊带：一种治疗压力性尿失禁的手术方式。在尿道中段下方放置一小段聚丙烯吊带。

不稳定性膀胱：患者的症状为不能"憋尿"（尿急）、白天经常上厕所（尿频）或晚上多次起床解尿（夜尿症）。

尿道：膀胱排空尿液经过的管道。

急迫性尿失禁：当有"必须去解手"的感觉时，还没来得及赶到厕所就尿湿了。

尿动力学：测量排尿时的膀胱压力和尿流率。

子宫脱垂：子宫下移至阴道内。

外阴痛：阴道口的疼痛或者烧灼感。

（上海交通大学医学院附属第六人民医院妇产科，薛卓维 译，张睿 校）

INDEX

索引

T

tethered vagina   78

TVT   40,42,172,184,186

U

urge incontinence   4,56,58,94,134,174,176

urinary incontinence   40,58,68,186

urodynamics   56,186

urodynamic testing   150

V

vulvodynia   82,92–98

（上海交通大学医学院附属第六人民医院　徐依赟　翻译　梁爽
校稿）

英文缩写词表

缩写	英文	中文	页码
A	anus	肛门	8,9
ATFP	arcus tendineus fascia pelvis	盆筋膜腱弓	146,147
BN	bladder neck	膀胱颈	80
CL	cardinal ligament	主韧带	146,147
CX	cervix	子宫颈	10,175
EUL	external urethral ligament	尿道外韧带	126,146,147
F	fascia	筋膜	127
FDA	Food and Drug Administration	食品药品监督管理局	39,67
FI	faecal incontinence	便失禁	4,43,52,66
H	suburethral vagina（hammock）	尿道下阴道（吊床）	2
HRT	Hormone replacement therapy	激素替代治疗	32,33
N	nerve endings/stretch receptors	神经末梢/牵张感受器	28,29
PB	perineal body	会阴体	10,11,24,25
PCF	pubocervical fascia	耻骨宫颈筋膜	146,147
PRM	puborectalis muscle	耻骨直肠肌	42,43
PUL	pubourethral ligament	耻骨尿道韧带	59,146,147
RVF	rectovaginal fascia	直肠阴道筋膜	146,147
R	rectum	直肠	7,8,10
S	sacrum	骶骨	8,9,38,39

SI	stress incontinence	压力性尿失禁	2,3,22,23
T	tapes	吊带	41,43,55
TVT	tension-free vaginal tape	无张力阴道吊带	187
TFS	tissue fixation system	组织固定系统（特定的手术器械和名称）	27,40,41
U	urethra	尿道	8,12,14
USL	uterosacral ligament	子宫骶骨韧带	146
UT	uterus	子宫	6,7,8,9
V	vagina	阴道	2,3,4,5